Pendulum

Unlock Your Inner Magic and Enhance Your Life

(How to Use Them for Divination, Dowsing, Tarot Reading, Healing, and Balancing Chakras)

Shane Burdett

Published By **John Kembrey**

Shane Burdett

Pendulum: Unlock Your Inner Magic and Enhance Your Life (How to Use Them for Divination, Dowsing, Tarot Reading, Healing, and Balancing Chakras)

ISBN 978-1-7388580-8-8

No part of this guidebook shall be reproduced in any form without permission in writing from the publisher except in the case of brief quotations embodied in critical articles or reviews.

Legal & Disclaimer

Table Of Contents

Chapter 1: Pendulum History and Its Origin

The History of the Pendulum

What Is a Pendulum? When and How Does It Arise?

Maybe in the end, you have stumble upon this unusual and unusual object known as a pendulum. If so, you've likely puzzled what it is and what it's used for. The pendulum is a small tool, commonly conical in shape, it without a doubt is suspended from a string.

Something to preserve in mind is that the duration of this string can range from one pendulum to each different. What is immovable is that the wire or chain need to live regular inside the tool; that is, it should neither stretch nor cut returned.

The pendulum is accountable for generating an oscillatory motion, additionally referred to as a periodic movement. In one of a kind words, it may flow into constantly and repetitively. Of path, effective elements at once have an effect on the pendulum's conduct, which incorporates the period of the string, the peak from which the pendulum is held, and the airspeed throughout the pendulum.

Origin of the Pendulum

The pendulum is an artifact that has been acknowledged for masses of years. Still, the first man to increase a scientific use for this device come to be Galileo Galilei, the Italian-born astronomer, physicist, mathematician, and fact seeker referred to as the father of contemporary astronomy.

Galileo Galilei have become born in Pisa, Italy, on February 15, 1564 AD. He revolutionized the area of era with its novel epistemological idea, laying the guidelines of current-day scientific research via along with in experiments and essays the classical rigor of the clinical method. This technique promoted the regular experimentation of the numerous natural phenomena that surrounded it.

According to what facts maintains and contemplates, inside the destiny, in 1583, Galilei decided how a lamp hung from the ceiling of the Cathedral of Pisa. It grow to be continuously shifting, and he observed out that the length of the movement did not alternate, even though the amplitude of the oscillation frequently decreased. This discovery changed into what gave starting to his experimentation. Galilei repeated the test over and over as a manner to have a take a look at and collate the effects. However, he did now not do it on my own; he desired the help of some companions to tie two rather heavy spheres to ropes of equal lengths, which they driven at exquisite distances.

They placed that the oscillations have been the equal in each pendulums in the same duration however constantly considered that the strings were the identical duration.

Thus, Galilei changed into capable of decide that the duration of the penculum's oscillation trusted the length of the string. Still, it became independent of the mass of the object on the stop of it. From the ones investigations, Isochronism have grow to be diagnosed, which refers back to the equality of duration in the movements of a frame, the oscillations of the pendulum, and the vibrations of a flywheel-spiral system.

From that discovery, severa scientists used the pendulum to carry out their investigations in extraordinary experiments. Isaac Newton become certainly one in every of them, having used it to calculate the consistent of the acceleration of gravity on Earth. Also, to determine the primary clear approximation of the velocity of sound to demonstrate the connection between mass and weight to refute the concept of the ether's existence and to observe the physical conduct of colliding gadgets.

Another wonderful scientist who used the pendulum in his experiments have come to be the Dutch astronomer, physicist, and mathematician Christian Huygens, who, in 1656, created the clock based completely absolutely at the pendulum.

The pendulum also completed a massive feature within the life of the famend astronomer

Jean-Bernard León Foucault, who, in 1851, used it to demonstrate the existence of the Earth's rotational movement, subsequently the term Foucault's Pendulum.

At present, the pendulum is used to degree time, plumbing, dowsing, detecting magnetic fields, and detecting energies. Still, some humans use it as an accurate method of divination right away related to technology.

Chapter 2: Classification

Types of Pendulums

Due to their basis, inclinations, and a couple of makes use of, we're able to decide a huge form of various pendulums. Since new pendulums seem through the years, it is probably now not viable to decide precisely what number of there are, but allow's take a better study these instruments.

The first ones were quite easy and consisted of a easy key suspended from a thread to which, even because it moved, questions were asked. Answers have been constrained to a certain or no. With the passage of time, rather than a key, a hoop or a small ball of lead have become used, but continuously with the same purpose.

Eventually, the pendulum acquired many more bureaucracy with the addition of aesthetic functions. You can see small crystalline spheres suspended from gold chains or conical pendulums in materials collectively with ebony or ivory.

Many diviners choose to use a strong quartz pendulum, regardless of the reality that they require consistent energetic cleansing due to the fact the pendulum can be extra with out hassle charged with all styles of negative or high-quality energies which can intrude with the give up cease end result.

For better precision, using an spherical and pointed pendulum is recommended. It want to additionally be requisite to tie a knot at each give up, from which the pendulum hangs, to save you it from slipping thru the arms.

Although there are brilliant pendulums, the entirety will rely upon you and which you experience you need to select. I endorse that you ponder this and choose out the only that your coronary heart dictates considering that this could be the only that offers you the proper solutions. A connection has to emerge amongst you and the pendulum. You will recognize it even as you see it due to the fact you'll feel an immediate courting on the way to tell you that that is your pendulum.

Let's test some of the most used pendulums:

Simple or Basic Pendulum

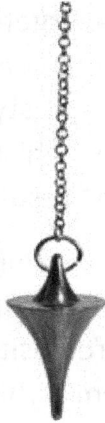

The clean pendulum is used as a reference to begin on the direction of divination and is for those individuals who need to start running in the direction of the artwork of feeling electricity. These pendulum are used for any diagnosis and are best for dowsing, an historical era used to remotely stumble on radiation emitted thru all people or any form of energy. Very a hit consequences are done when utilized in combination with Reiki remedies, among others.

Isis Pendulum of four, 6, 9, or 16 Batteries

The Isis Pendulum is one of the maximum well-known, appreciated, and used Egyptian pendulums. It has a high dowsing sensitivity and sends further to receives strength. Its 4, 6, nine, or 12 batteries allow balancing radiation, and the greater batteries it has, the extra powerful it is. It is of top notch dowsing sensitivity and is specifically liable for reestablishing the lack of strength for physical improvement.

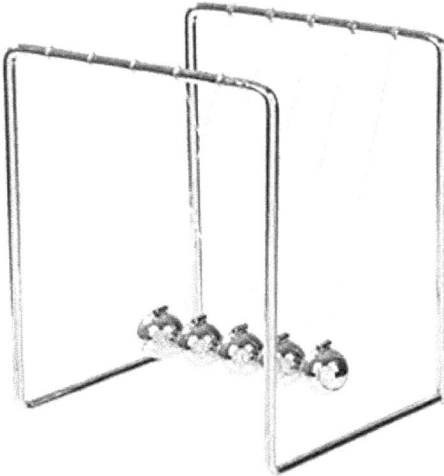

Newton's pendulum

Newton's Pendulum is an tool composed of 5 same balls, every considered one of which hangs from a body with the aid of threads of identical duration so that all of them are in contact and aligned. When one of the balls is separated from one stop, allowing it to collide with the others, the ball at the other cease starts offevolved shifting and reaches the equal pinnacle because of the truth the ball to begin with released. At the same time, the rest of the balls stay at rest.

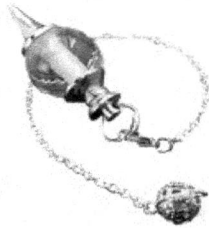

Foucault Pendulum

The Foucault pendulum have come to be introduced in 1851 with the aid of French physicist Léon Foucault and conceived as an take a look at to illustrate the Earth's rotation. It is a spherical pendulum that might swing freely in any vertical aircraft and can achieve this for severa hours.

The Foucault Pendulum is usually used to demonstrate the rotation of the Earth.

Ballistic Pendulum

This is a tool that allows for the dedication of the velocity of a projectile. This pendulum is made from a massive block of mass wood, suspended thru two vertical threads, and a bullet is fired horizontally toward a block suspended from a rope. This tool is called a ballistic pendulum, it's miles used to decide the bullet's pace through using measur ng the attitude the pendulum deflects after the bullet has embedded itself in it.

Torsion Pendulum

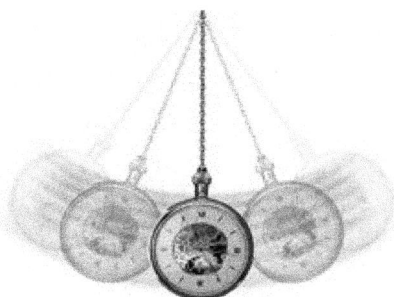

This pendulum is an object with oscillations due to rotation spherical an axis through the pendulum. It lets in you to discover each damped oscillations and compelled adjustments. In different phrases, the torsion pendulum includes a vertically suspended spherical drift-phase of cord, with its higher surrender ordinary. From the lower give up hangs a frame with a known or available to calculate the at once of inertia. Any movement can be decomposed as a aggregate of linear and rotational movements.

Osiris Pendulum

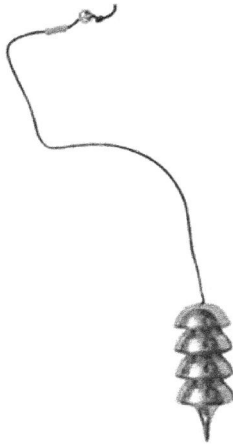

The Osiris Pendulum belongs to the gathering of Egyptian pendulums. It has a fantastic energetic strength because of its geometric shape, and it is made from four over apping hemispheres. The first has a peaked drop, and the others twist one over the opposite. This pendulum's strong point is that it eliminates poor energies. It need to be used for viral and bacterial remedies, therefore doing away with them from the frame.

Telluric Pendulum

This Pendulum has a format organized as a manner to capture all sorts of telluric and cosmic radiation. Exceptional artwork is being finished in houses and places of work to locate geographically affected areas.

UFO Pendulum

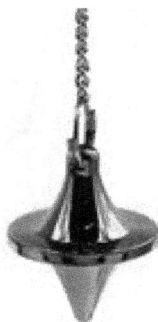

This pendulum serves to seize the re-emission of dowsing energies. It is used specially for power diagnostics and remedies and unique dowsing art work that consists of searching out groundwater, lacking oldsters, and extraordinary minerals.

Atlantean pendulum

This pendulum has notable functionality and is generally encouraged for novices and specialists alike. This pendulum has an precise precision in its evaluation; it receives rid of poor thoughts, is a amazing personal protector, and allows regain out of place intellectual energy.

Bronze Karnak Pendulum

There is a replica of this pendulum placed in a sarcophagus within the Valley of the Kirgs.

This pendulum is suitable for any dowsing and tele-dowsing work and works with a long way flung and intellectual work. It moreover has the particularity of being a excellent wave emitter. Its energy acts via its elongated and have come to be form. This is one of the maximum used pendulums in dowsing and restoration practices.

Karnak Quartz Pendulum

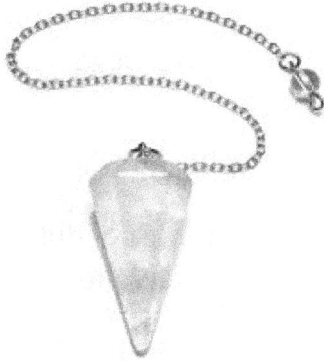

The functions that quartz possesses are mixed with this pendulum's houses given thru its famous shape. Thanks to its balanced curvature, this historic pendulum radiates its energy, making it possible for use as a transmitter and receiver. It is a suitable pendulum for each the amateur and the professional dowser.

Due to its sensitivity and accuracy, it is able to be used for a huge style of applications. Quartz offers it notable functionality thinking about it's far the most powerful strength amplifier in the world. It has recuperation homes, generates electromagnetism, and dissipates static strength.

Witness Pendulum

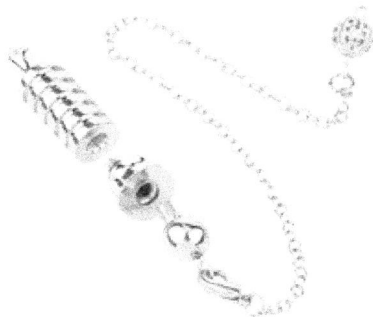

This pendulum is crafted from separate factors: body and lid. It is a pendulum that is easy to deal with and surely beneficial, with exceptional precision due to its extremely good stability and weight. It additionally possesses woman power. There is a small hollow space within the pendulum that permits the place of witness material to manual the studying better. This kind of pendulum is indicated in strength work taught at distances or for readings wherein it's far critical to enhance the vibrations with a particular fabric.

Wooden Pendulum

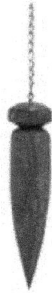

Some pick the timber pendulum because of the fact, being a unbiased fabric, it isn't always suffering from electromagnetic fields, and the solution is typically greater accurate. After using this pendulum kind, it want to be de-impregnated with a mild blow in competition to a robust floor.

Rod of Power Pendulum

These rod-fashioned strength pendulums function a quartz and crystal spike and sphere. They are considerably advocated pendulums to diploma the chakras' power and, to be used alongside side Reiki techniques, can also be utilized in dowsing and any consultation or strength length. Each one is a totally particular piece, and the irregularities inside the end of every pendulum do not constitute defects but as an alternative an average exceptional of Hindu handicrafts.

Bronze Spiral Pendulum

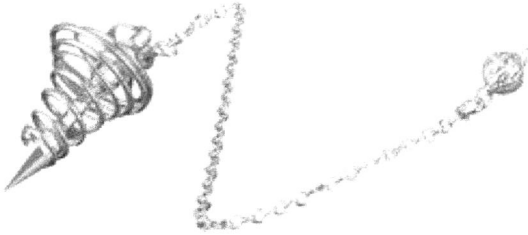

This spiral-fashioned pendulum is utilized in remedy as an aspirator of energies that overload the affected vicinity. It has an good sized ability to absorb power.

Merkaba Pendulum

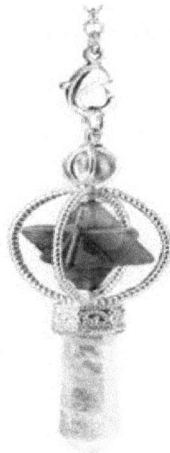

This pendulum is accountable for growing and integrating awareness as it allows interdimensional displacement and aligns the systems that make up the individual. It takes the shape of a movie star fabricated from opposing tetrahedra in region; one elements up and the alternative down. Symbolically, one in every of its angles elements to Heaven and some other to Earth. The characteristic that makes this pendulum a superb tool is that it appeals to the electricity because of a rotation in the contrary course of each tetrahedron.

Semiprecious Stones Pendulum

This pendulum is made with noble semi-precious stones. Besides being splendid pendulums for session, moreover they include the specific houses of rocks. Lapis lazuli colour stimulates instinct, black tourmaline neutralizes bad energies, and the tiger's eye favors the release of electricity the least bit ranges.

Chacras Stones Pendulum

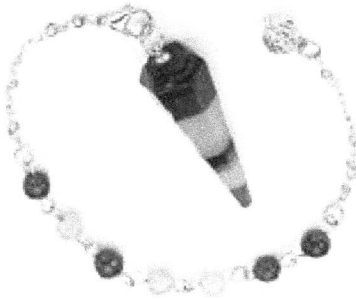

This pendulum is quite powerful for electricity restoration and can be discovered in triangular, round, and polyhedron shapes. The outstanding geometric shapes paintings with fantastic styles of energies depending on every person. This pendulum is crafted from seven stones of diverse hues associated with the chakras constant with their respective colors. These stones select the consultation or analysis made with the pendulum, making the solutions and effects greater real.

Rose Quartz Pendulum

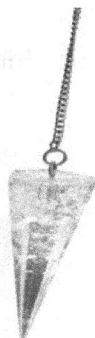

The purple color of this pendulum is because of its titanium content material fabric. Quartz is taken into consideration the stone of the coronary coronary heart, and it opens and strengthens the fourth chakra, connecting with the affection of oneself and the affection of the universe. It also connects with internal peace, encouraging non-public fulfillment. It is a useful restoration stone that allows you to release the repressed feelings within the coronary heart. It promotes friendship, love, and harmony. It may be very suitable for kids, due to its softness and surprise.

White Quartz Pendulum

Shamanic traditions keep in mind white quartz a stone of mild, cognizance, and clairvoyance. This pendulum cleans and balances highbrow, non secular, and emotional energies. It generates and transmits first-class power while repelling and transmuting bad strength. It has resonant residences, balances the air of mystery, and allows inside the remedy of any illness. It is related to the seventh chakra however may be utilized in some different middle to help empower, channel, or perhaps balance power. It favors the reference to the interior mild and is considered an amplifier and enhancer, so it's miles critical to be well-focused on the identical time as the use of it.

Green Quartz Pendulum

Green quartz is a mild stone of harmony and renewal. It is considered a stone of properly-being and prosperity and offers a balance among mind and body, imparting balance and emotional calmness. It is ideally used within the coronary heart chakra to unblock it and promote its regeneration. A green quartz pendulum is typically used as an anti inflammatory for recovery pores and skin and eye ailments.

Agate Pendulum

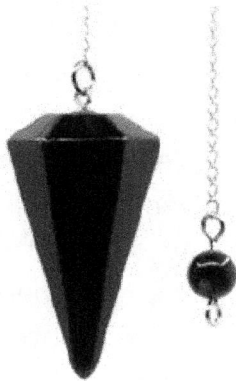

Agate is a microcrystalline sort of the quartz group. There are many types of agates, and their shade relies upon at the most effective of a type materials they will comprise. The maximum sufficient are the gray variety. Agate is considered a gentle electricity stone appeared for bringing concord and balance. It fosters self-self guarantee and cognizance, similarly to promotes non secular growth, love, and courage. Placing this pendulum at the brow calms fever and complications, and at the same time as placed alongside the legs, allows to get rid of retained fluids. The agate pendulum generally enhances restoration electricity.

Lunar Pendulum completed

Moonstone is a stone of internal growth and strength that soothes emotional instability and stress, enhances instinct, and promotes idea, fulfillment, and accurate fortune in love and business corporation topics. This pendulum promotes balance, calm, and peace. Placed on the solar plexus, it helps to generate a strong balance. It represents the cyclical nature of the man or woman or women and favors emotional, mental, and physical stability in internal boom processes. It is considered a religious stone, and it empowers the Ying a part of human beings. It furthermore promotes the steadiness among masculine and female energies.

Additionally, moonstone can gain the woman reproductive cycle, alleviate period-related illnesses, and balance the hormonal machine. This stone is related to the Third Eye Chakra and Solar Plexus Chakra. You can discover them in one-of-a-kind sunglasses, like pink, cream, yellow, blue or grey.

Amethyst Pendulum

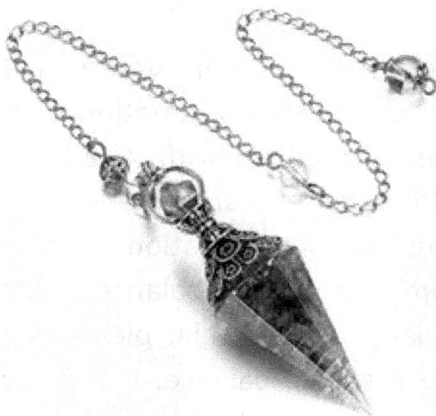

Amethyst is a number of quartz of magmatic and hydrothermal foundation. Its violet shade is due to its iron oxide content mater al and the excessive temperatures it is subjected to inside the route of its formation. It is one of the first gemstones implemented in historic instances as an ornamental stone and a symbol of wealth and power. It moreover knows the manner to be related with purity and spirituality.

Amethyst is known as the stone of harmony, transmutation, and spirituality. It corresponds to the 6th chakra, that is positioned some of the eyebrows. It helps to calm the mind, for this reason promoting the connection with intuition. For this cause, amethyst is commonly an superb complement to the workout of meditation. This may be done with the resource of protecting the mineral on your arms, setting it above the forehead or coronary heart, or putting an amethyst crystal in the front of you at some stage in your exercise.

Tiger Eye Pendulum

This pendulum is severa quartz with a feature yellow and brown shade that has a reflective optical effect that resembles the eye of a feline. The tiger's eye is taken into consideration a stone associated with creativity, energy, and stability. It is idea to be the union of the power of the solar and that of the Earth. It is taken into consideration a protective stone that favors rooting, and also can enhance one's vanity and mood. Additionally, the tiger's eye is often related to prosperity.

Tree of Life Pendulum

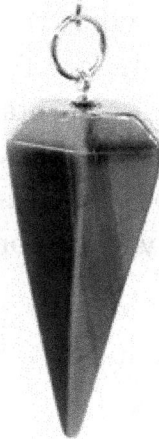

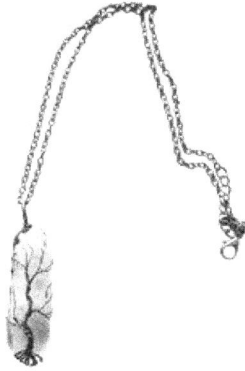

The tree of lifestyles has been used worldwide for centuries, representing the interconnection among all existence on our planet. It has been visible as a sacred image, which consists of massive meanings in every non secular and religious philosophies global. Some cultures hold in mind it to be the tree of enlightenment, the tree of immortality, the supply of everlasting existence. For others, Buddha reached enlightenment under this tree, so it's far visible as a very sacred image.

Chapter 3: Use, Operation, Consecration of the Pendulum and Recommendations

The Use of the Pendulum and How it Works.

Many times, all we want is a unmarried technique to trade our lives definitely.

As we formerly installed, the area is complete of humans capable of inventing an unsure or maybe tragic destiny to accumulate coins in move lower back. They do not care to are seeking out for the fact, however human beings pays for it, although it is an invented truth.

If you knew a manner to use the pendulum your self, you may ask any questions you wanted and get the proper solutions. By this, I do no longer suggest which you will become a medium from one second to the subsequent, but that it'll direct you on the right path. You will apprehend that there's no person within the center with hidden pursuits: simply you and the reality of the pendulum.

For example, in case you suspect that someone is running witchcraft on you, you can ask your pendulum. If your pendulum answers positive, you have to ask who it's miles, citing the names of human beirgs you agree with you studied are suspicious. You also can ask which character you need to visit verify this and cleanse you of that witchcraft. The pendulum will restriction itself to answering affirmatively or negatively. If the answer is "no," which you need to not go to that character. The solutions want to guide you until they lead you to the proper person.

Cleaning and Consecration of the Pendulum

Whether living or inanimate, every being harbors all forms of power: exceptional, horrible, or impartial. As we do no longer recognize how many people have touched a modern pendulum, it is able to be loaded with many fantastic energies. After all, the manner of the pendulum is exactly to build up the power of human beings.

There are brilliant processes to smooth the pendulum, so I will show you the maximum not unusual way to smooth your pendulum. Of route, before seeing to the cleansing of the pendulum, you need to undergo in thoughts that it's far essential first to consecrate it so that, after cleansing, it can cross again to its primary energy country.

The first step is to thank the spirit that lives in the pendulum. You need to ask its permission to apply it for your gain and the gain of others.

Follow the instructions under:

Draw a circle with chalk at the ground and location it inner with the four elements: air, fireplace, earth, and water. I use incense for air, a white candle for the fireside, a tumbler of water for water, and a chunk dust in a small field for the earth. Say, "I consecrate this pendulum with the electricity of air, hearth, earth, and water. With the blessing of our heavenly father and with the assist of all of the ones beings of mild that accompany me, you will be used for appropriate constant with my will, to advocate and help anyone who comes to me requesting assist".

Hold the pendulum and say, "By the electricity of the four elements" earlier than passing the pendulum over the incense and announcing, "By the power of the air." Continue passing the pendulum over the lit candle, pronouncing, "By the strength of the fireplace." Then sprinkle the pendulum with water, pronouncing "purified by way of manner of manner of water." Finally, immerse the pendulum in the soil, announcing, "Empowered via the energy of the earth."

Place the pendulum amongst your hands and blow your breath lightly so that you begin to create a proper away reference to your pendulum. Do this for at the least minutes, pay attention, meditate and ask for clarity, fantastic strength, and plenty of benefits to transmit the message correctly. Ask your beings of slight to enlighten you and promise to continuously work for the energy of mild and do real for others. With this, you can consecrate your pendulum and consequently collect a determination to use its electricity for your self and whoever involves you for useful resource. The extremely good time to consecrate the pendulum is among 6:00 AM and 9:00 AM because of the fact the strength may be purest.

After the incense and candle were honestly fed on, the pendulum might be consecrated. You can use it straight away or preserve it in its right vicinity. You ought to no longer permit honestly every body to touch it. If this takes area, you want to smooth it another time, as it may accumulate horrific energies—it is pleasant to learn how to clean it well.

How do you smooth it? It could be first-rate if you put together a field with a tablespoon of sea salt, area the pendulum internal and allow it soak in the solution for an afternoon. If the object is hooked up to a silver chain, you may want to put off it due to the fact the salt can motive some damage. If the pendulum has any steel additives, get rid of those because the salt may additionally oxidize them.

After this time, you may put off the pendulum from the box and allow it dry. You will take the pendulum outdoor to achieve the solar's rays for multiple hours. After a few hours, your pendulum can be equipped. You will vicinity it inside the palm of your hand and placed your different hand on top to transmit your power. You also can blow air onto the pendulum to exchange your power.

Another manner is to go away it sitting on a selenite stone, as that could be a powerful electricity cleaner.

Another way to smooth it consists of the elements of water, earth, air, and hearth. We will bypass the pendulum thru every of the factors as we are announcing the subsequent sentences and for each;

Air detail, I invoke you to provide us speed and intellectual freedom. The water element, I invoke you to supply us love and creativity. Element fire, I invoke you to bless us together with your purification.

Earth detail, I invoke you to grant us power, stability, and protection. I claim you, winds of intelligence, to fill our lives with understanding.

And so that you permit us to apply purpose with out negative the instinct and as a end result open our minds to recognition and clearing all doubts.

Recommendations for Using the Pendulum

Before using your pendulum, you want to discover a quiet region in your house wherein you could pay interest and now not using a noise or distractions of any type. This may be in a nook in your private home in which you region a small table, or perhaps take a seat at the ground. I select out a desk to speak about with the pendulum. On the desk, I surely have the photograph of Saint Michael alongside white and crimson candles. I moreover use stones, like white quartz and incense. You can embody any object that has non secular fee to you.

I artwork with angels, so I invoke my determine angel, however that is a non-public preference. It all is based upon on what works best for you. You will understand this due to the reality you may enjoy inexplicable electricity and recognize which pendulum you must pick.

Protection should moreover be considered. There are many techniques to do this, and of direction, actually everyone adapts to the fine manner to do it consistent with their very personal ideals and religion. After all, it does not paintings within the equal way for anybody. If you note that some issue isn't always walking for you, it is able to be due to the truth your location and intellectual location aren't as ordered as they should be for you. It is critical to artwork resultseasily at the equal time as respecting your very very very own beliefs. Forcing subjects will cause now not anything.

Using the pendulum is quite clean, but it takes attention and exercise, that's normally the maximum difficult factor to get started out.

When asking our pendulum a query about our destiny, the unconscious responds through spherical motions on the object. The pendulum will accentuate these moves and be directed in a specific path, indicating an affirmative or negative solution.

You need to put the pendulum five centimeters from your hand, which must now not be demanding, to obtain this solution. The palm of your hand, in flip, needs to be directed in the route of the sky.

In a cushty u . S . A ., you can ask the pendulum to inform you a "Yes" and a "No" so that you understand the end stop result of your questions; all pendulums are high-quality, and therefore the way they solution moreover varies. You should additionally ask if you can perform the question consultation. Then preserve excellent on the same time as you purchased an affirmative solution.

When you ask the query, the pendulum will start to swing through answering yes or no. The direction in which it swings or aspect to side will answer the query. You need to instinctively realise the "no" is and the "yes" of your pendulum whilst you see them. Once the "no" and the "positive" were recognized, it's going to constantly be the equal motion.

It is possible that, after the number one movement, the pendulum will make a exquisite one. When it makes a motion and then makes a super or possibly contradictory one a few seconds later, it can advocate that the statistics supplied corresponds to two extremely good levels or conditions. It might be that there is a couple of accurate answer or that it is greater complicated than it seems. If so, you need to trade your question to be greater precise one and obtain facts for the two conditions.

The pendulum does not lie or misinform, however it may on occasion have many solutions. This can cause confusion. Either way, take it clean! There is constantly a way to smooth maximum of these doubts, so if you aren't positive of the answer that's been provided ask the pendulum if it's far telling you the whole fact. Then ask if you may ask the same question once more. If the solution is the identical both times, it is due to the reality it is a specific fact.

Something that you want to no longer ignore at any time is your intuition thru the pendulum, as it will advise you on what your frame and thoughts want most for his or her accurate evolution.

The possibilities are endless. Once you have found out to understand the pendulum's use, it's going to probably be a expertise you can take with you anywhere and characteristic available while you want it.

What you have to in no manner forestall keeping in mind is why you operate the pendulum. It isn't always actually beneficial to deviate from the direction of pinnacle or use it as a game to ponder special options. This is because of the reality it can redecorate into a few difficulty very horrific now not handiest for the life of the person who is coming to you but moreover for you. Using the pendulum is sacred; notable in case you are inclined to recognize it will you be capable of use it and be successful within the future.

Chapter 4: Dowsing

Connection with Divination

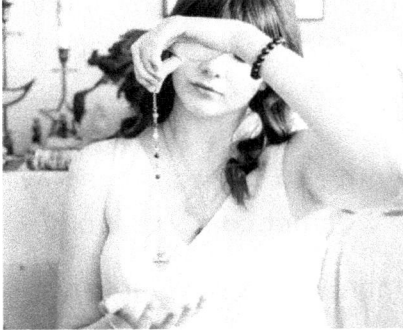

How Is Dowsing Linked to Divination?

Dowsing is a totally ancient technclogical knowledge used, every at that issue and nowadays, to discover the radiation emitted thru any form of energy.

Different peoples of the world use this technique to look for groundwater, minerals, and oil. In more contemporary times, dowsing have been used to search for misplaced items, lacking humans, and extraordinary divinatory techniques. The devices maximum used for dowsing are the pendulum, rotating metallic rods, and dowsing rods.

The body captures, amongst distinct vibrations, the precise colors of mild strength and the particular tones of sound strength, each of which vibrates at a selected frequency. These perceptions, but, are not carried out entirely via the organs of sight or being attentive to due to the fact we feel and anticipate with our complete body.

Some human beings have advanced the right mind greater efficaciously. These are those who have the innate capability to dowse and gain fulfillment in the are seeking. However, no matter this gain, dowsing is a era that ought to be positioned and requires recognition, schooling, and perseverance to be completely mastered.

Training to comprehend dowsing takes time and staying strength so it could be performed with will and care. With this completed, we're able to seize the radiation emitted through manner of ourselves and the our our bodies and forms of electricity surrounding us.

As for the electricity of the pendulum, it has programs in all fields of existence, at the same time as the improvement of the potential to apply dowsing is beneficial for any selection we want to make. Using our instinct via dowsing allows us to boom functions we are able to use to make any desire.

However, this is not a few component that most effective fortune-tellers or psychics exercise. Many docs use the pendu um to diagnose diseases and their motives and decide suitable treatments, tablets, duration of treatments, and the frequency and dose with which effective medicinal drugs need to be administered.

Pendulum dowsing is an alternative medication technique supposed to be used for analysis and is carefully related to the fields defined thru acupuncture. A well-known application of dowsing, probable the best with the longest culture, is finished with the aid of using the so-called dowsers who claim with the intention to discover the most favorable websites for the excavation of wells, wherein the water desk is greater handy.

Although a few take this workout as a few thing out of date, the meant makes use of of dowsing are diverse and had been executed as a particular era given that historic instances.

Dowsing can:

- Diagnose sicknesses

- Obtain actual measurements

- Find water

- Find minerals

- Predict modern-day or destiny states of residing depend

- Find lost gadgets

- Locate electricity radiation factors

- Find humans

- Guess numbers and combinations

Chapter 5: The History of the Celtic Cross and Symbolism

When Did the Celtic Cross Arise? What Does It Symbolize?

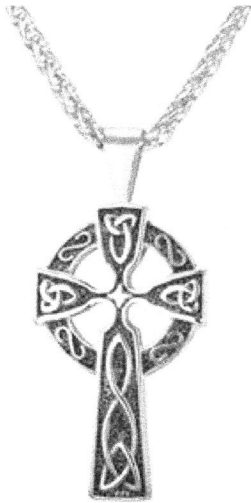

Throughout data, humanity has been characterised with the beneficial useful resource of the arrival of devices with particular symbolisms, to which a vast spiritual, spiritual and cultural load is attributed. In many instances, these symbols outline the interaction among human beings of a specific region and lifestyle.

One of those symbols is the Celtic skip, being one of the oldest of humanity. From the way it appears, the traditional Christian skip converges next to the wheel, it truly is why some suppose it could be derived from the solar wheel. However, in assessment to the sun wheel, the four ends of the bypass protrude outside the circle.

The Celtic pass is one of the maximum not unusual and famous Celtic symbols and has huge cultural and spiritual importance. It is not anything however a petroglyph originating from the ancient Celtic peoples of Great Britain, Ireland, and France.

Various theories provide an reason for its foundation, however because the Celtic way of life become transmitted first-rate orally, it is no longer viable to verify any as specific and accurate.

Due to its similarity to the Christian bypass, the Celtic pass is also used by believers in this faith, notwithstanding the reality that its statistics originates prolonged earlier than Christianity even existed. The Celtic move is a spiritual picture of the historical Celtic people, whose origins date again to the 7th century, starting the Christian era.

During the seventh century, the Celtic cross became engraved on huge stones placed on the floor, and later embellished Christian churches or temples in Great Britain, Scotland, and Ireland.

There are variously historical, religious, non secular, and esoteric interpretations of the meaning of the Celtic flow. The ends of the circulate out of doors the circle represent the 4 elements: water, air, earth, and fireside. On the opposite side, it represents north, south, east, and west.

The union of the that means of the four factors in the equal photo is recurrent in Celtic lifestyle and different symbols, together with the triskele, triquetra, and sun skip.

When we study the Celtic pass, we are able to recognize that each one 4 arms are the equal. That is why people who devote themselves to the research of symbolism maintain that this option shows the choice of guy to recognize himself and his challenge in life, even as, thru it, he manages to specific 4 channels to reap ascension: the popularity of "I," nature, recognition, and God. This way that, in the Celtic skip, special types of sacred energies converge that invite us to go beyond harmoniously at the same time as our transit thru the universe takes region.

Because each stop of the Celtic glide symbolizes better energy that unites one to the opportunity through an wonderful circle concurrently intersecting in a common center, the transcendence of it will lie in the reputation of our origin. Unique and religious in communion with the sacred.

Because of these beliefs, the Celtic pass is taken into consideration a conjunction of hopeful factors of existence, wherein honor, faith, balance, and harmony create the appropriate stability to transcend to a higher global.

In different terms, respecting the symbolism of the Celtic flow into as a guiding element ensures that it'll take us correctly via our existence, recognizing ourselves as non secular beings in transit toward a higher and better destination.

For the Celts and thinking about the four factors that unite and be a part of, developing a bridge among divine energies and man, the cross has the equal symbolic association because the Tree of Life. It have turn out to be also the symbol of the 4 seasonal fairs that marked the Celtic twelve months:

•Imbolc: February 1, in which the awakening of nature and the earth's fertility is widely recognized, calling for achievement in future obligations.

•Beltane: May 1, at the same time as the virility of the gods is woke up, and for fertility.

•Lughnasadh: August 1, in which the start of the harvest festivities are celebrated, fruits are accumulated, and the blessing of the flocks is asked.

•Samhain: October 31, where the closing competition and the closing harvest of the 12 months are celebrated, moreover the give up of the cycle of the Celtic wheel.

The crosses made for the ones one-of-a-type sports had been adorned with drawings and figures common of Celtic artwork. In the earliest, engravings and geometric designs have been conventional of artwork in the British Isles. Still, from the 9th and 10th centuries, in addition they appear in symbolic representations of biblical scenes.

These crosses are referred to as Scripture crosses, and their complexity is such that they've emerge as described as "sermons in stone." The ornaments or knots indoors them represent infinity. Each of the recommendations marked with the aid of manner of the pass is also related, with the corresponding deity for each one just so it might be some element like this:

•East: God Lugh is associated with the air and gives safety together with his spear.

•South: Goddess Nuada, associated with hearth and whose sword made her a defender of feelings.

•West: God Dagda, related to water, covered and controlled the thoughts and idea.

•North: Seat of the Stone of Destiny L'a Fáil, the Stone of Tara, positive to the earth in which exceptional the rightful kings are crowned and accepted with the resource of the Druid gods.

Chapter 6: Other Celtic Symbols

Classification and Its Parts

How Are Celtic Symbols Understood?

Celtic symbols are immediately related to the mythology developed via Celtic peoples throughout the Iron Age. These peoples inhabited the islands of Great Britain and Ireland, amongst particular areas of Europe.

The Celtic peoples practiced the usage of diverse variations of Celtic languages and had polytheistic mythology. Most of those peoples maintained touch with the Roman Empire, such quite some abandoned their proper Celtic language and transformed to Christianity.

A massive part of Celtic mythology evolved even before the discovery of writing, that is why few written resources without delay describe the traditions of Celtic mythology. The beliefs of Celtic mythology had been specially transmitted orally at some point of its beginnings so there may be no documented proof.

What allowed us to construct a part of Celtic mythology are the symbols positioned and the writings and manuscripts of Greek and Roman authors knowledgeable of Celtic mythology.

We will check some of those symbols and their meanings.

Triquetra

The photo of the triquetra was constructed from 3 arches in the form of a triangle. The phrase triquetra comes from the Latin triquetrous, this means that "3 corners," subsequently its triangular shape. One of its peculiarities is that it seldom seems completely on my own in the portions of Celtic artwork that have resurfaced over time. This may additionally furthermore propose that it did now not typically have a due to this within Celtic mythology but as a substitute have become decorative. Due to its 3-element nature, this photo relates to Saint Patrick's shamrock, representing the trinity.

Triskele

The triskele or triskelion, moreover referred to as triple spiral, is a Celtic photo that includes three spirals joined in a triangular arrangement. The phrase triskelion comes from the Greek τρισκέλιον and manner "three-legged."

This Celtic photo has been interpreted in exceptional strategies, but they all have a deep dating with the importance of the big range three. In this manner, it is feasible to apprehend this image representing the beyond, the existing, and the destiny. The triskelion is referred to as a photograph of start, existence, and death.

Tree of Life

The tree of existence is one of the maximum important Celtic symbols, as it has generally been a imperative element of Celtic mythology. Trees usually had wonderful significance thinking about Celtic peoples believed they had been the ancestors of guys. For the Celtic peoples, wood were the supply of existence due to the truth they gave their stop result to feed themselves and have been corporations of steady haven.

One of the possible meanings of the image of the tree of life is that it represents the concord a few of the forces of nature to offer rise to existence. In addition, it is also possible to relate it to strength and information.

The Celts taken into consideration the natural cycle of bushes because of the 12 months's seasons, regarding it to loss of life in the direction of wintry weather and rebirth for the duration of spring. For the Celts, it grow to be so symbolic that they even planted a tree inside the center of every new agreement as a picture of existence.

Celtic Knots

The knots are mainly ornamental, used as ornamental motifs. Many of them appear engraved in stone or manuscripts from the Christian generation. The knots are depicted in the shape of braiding. In unique phrases, the photo indicates how the specific fragments of the tape intertwine, passing on occasion above and every now and then underneath. Also, Celtic knots don't have any stop, so the ribbon closes on itself.

There is an fantastic type of Celtic knots, and in loads of cases, it isn't feasible to give them a that means for the reason that they often have a really ornamental characteristic. It is viable that a number of these knots had a concrete which means that inside the beyond, but in maximum instances, this knowledge has been out of place because of the shortage of written transmission. Of direction, it should also be borne in mind that occasionally the precise which means that evolves, so it may even surely exchange during the Christianization of the Celtic peoples.

Celtic quaternary knot

The Celtic quaternary knot, additionally referred to as the defend knot, is one of the most vital and maximum taken into consideration Celtic knots. Its branch of a circle depicts it as four sections, which offers upward thrust to unique interpretations. On the only hand, the 4 sections of the ring can constitute the four number one factors. They can also represent the 4 sections because the four terrestrial tips or due to the fact the four seasons of the year.

One of the most sizable interpretations relates this knot to a defend, this is considered a photograph of protection.

Simple Spiral

The spiral is a recurring motif among Celtic symbols. There are many interpretations for the spiral signal, and experts declare that it's far a picture that represents the cycle of life: beginning, boom, and loss of lifestyles. The spiral photo moreover appears in special characters including the triskele, shaped through 3 spirals, or the systrel, original via circles.

Chapter 7: Operation and Use of the Celtic Cross, Magic and Tarot

Functioning and use of the Celtic Cross

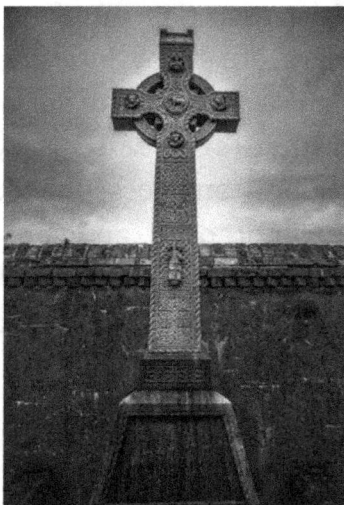

How Does the Celtic Cross Work?

We can say successfully that, in any trouble, the Celtic cross has usually been a picture of protection.

One of the maximum extensively taken into consideration theories is the advanced derivation of the sun wheel, which changed into crucial for its protective strength in opposition to witchcraft.

If we check with the pagans' view, the Celtic bypass photograph became understood as a mixture of figures: the electricity of the moon and the sun. The moon have become represented thru the circle, on the equal time because the power of the solar have grow to be conveyed via the bypass. The moon is generally related to the woman and the sun with the masculine. Many historians and university university college students of symbolism take transport of as genuine with that the Celtic pass represents the union of those additives.

The Celtic move is an icon whose because of this that and symbolism are carefully related to the inheritance of primitive pagan symbols, which refers back to the early tiers of Christianity and the adoption of this picture. There are a protracted way-proper companies these days who use this skip as a symbol of rejection of the present day-day religion.

Not simplest does it have those uses, but it's also associated with many different pagan landscapes, testimonies, creatures, and legends that talk of goblins, nymphs, fairies, and extremely good magical beings.

The Celtic move is a non secular, spiritual, and cultural photograph regularly utilized in sacred regions which include temples, cemeteries, and church homes.

Still, if there is a few element with which a direct connection has been generated is the Celtic flow, used as an object of protection, health, and authentic achievement.

It isn't uncommon to look at this flow into often used as a non secular protection amulet in competition to risky energies and, simultaneously, a compass a great way to allow one to light up the direction of nicely in our lives. Although the Celtic bypass is used as an amulet for believers and practitioners of magic, it's miles a image for steering to the greater great. It can be placed and utilized in severa methods.

Many choose out to place on rings collectively with waft charms. Some have spikes on their hands, braids, or gadgets with runes inner, gems, or valuable stones on their recommendations.

Some choose out tattoos. Due to the top notch power and symbolism of the Celtic cross indicates, wearing it at the pores and pores and skin has additionally turn out to be a fashion among those new fans of Celtic manner of existence. It continuously has the equal that means: protection and steerage in the direction of suitable with distinct paperwork and further data.

It has even been visible in trademarks of a huge variety. This picture may be decided hidden or positioned in a completely discreet way to encompass a few magic. If we look intently, we are able to find it discovered in numerous emblems of each day use, searching for to transport disregarded. These symbolize electricity and magic for folks who use them.

Some diviners pick out the bypass as their number one device because of its guiding talents and the intense energies it handles, combining the reason of the divinatory with the strength of the Celtic skip, developing a harmonic union to be used as an element of divination in human beings. This pendulum may be very powerful because of the fact, in addition to channeling the energies, it guarantees safety and leads the man or woman on an extremely good, safe, and religious direction.

With this effective symbology in thoughts, many supply a Celtic flow into amulet for considered one of a type reasons. In its Druid or Christian versions, everyone will employ the symbolism and power that fantastic fits their beliefs, which encompass safety, achievement, concord, and different meanings.

Wearing the Celtic skip as an amulet, in a few thing manner or for the motive you need, will provide you with help and safety at the route you pick out in existence.

The Celtic Cross, Its Magic, and the Tarot

The use of the Celtic circulate in magic is proper now associated with the use of Tarot Cards. This form of card reading allows you to refine the results to get more specific and reliable facts approximately the questions you have for your mind. This form of magic will permit one to get solutions and possibilities approximately the near and faraway future.

You receives the right feature of the spread and its interpretation, then with it, the possibilities you are looking for to take a look at your route and trade route. Meditate at the alternatives you are making to your lifestyles.

The Celtic waft has four paths that intersect. What you need to do is pick out considered considered one in all them. This is a selection that is predicated upon completely on you.

The Celtic move is one of the oldest and most entire units of cards in tarot. Each position is set up with others, representing a selected state of affairs seen from the prevailing 2nd. Composed of ten gambling cards, those display the improvement of a hassle dynamically.

Let's see the this means that of the positions:

• Situation. Letter with the primary undertaking depend. What 's taking place?

• How is the state of affairs expressed?

• Trigger. Deeper desires.

• Where will we come from?. Past. We lived it till then.

• Objective. What we want to acquire. What are we looking beforehand to?.

• Where are we going? The destiny. What is ready to take vicinity?

• We. How does what takes place affects us?

• How do others apprehend us? How do they feel approximately us?

• Expectations. What we worry and what we preference.

• Consequences. Where is the state of affairs going?

Interactions amongst positions:

Position 1 is in which the studying is centered. It represents the primary electricity that defines the real state of affairs; it is its base.

Know that this card represents the solution on your query. The distinct positions of the playing cards tell the story; why is that this going on?

Where is it going? What is likely to take area next, how do you deal with the scenario, and what manifests consequently?

(Positions 1, 3 and 5) vs Temporal state of affairs (Positions four, 2 and 6)

Positions 1, three, and five constitute the prevailing, which will be the essential and modern-day second of the situation. The card in function 1 is the coronary coronary heart. The card in role 5 represents our notion, how we see it. The card in function 3 represents our unconscious motivation.

Positions 2, 4, and 6 constitute the temporal state of affairs, wherein we come from, and wherein we are going. The card in function 2 suggests the impact we are managing and what we're going thru inside the present. The card in position four suggests what's behind us, the beyond, and what we've got were given got professional. The card in function 6 indicates what is coming within the instant future and the way it needs to be addressed.

The Road to Conclusion (Positions 7, eight, 9 and 10)

The card in characteristic 7 shows us our attitude, at the same time as function 8 suggests how our surroundings perceives us. Position 9 represents expectancies, which can be what are conditioning our mindsets. The conjunction of all of these is seen in function 10, because of this the outcome of our actions.

Expectations (Position nine)

Expectations are represented thru the cardboard that falls in position nine. These expectancies that seem concerning the primary trouble rise up from beyond reports. The card in feature 9 is the maximum critical card after the card in function one, because it conditions our perspective. We may additionally additionally even find out information of ways we method the past.

Consequences (Position 10)

Position 10 represents the effects that the situation creates in our lives. It way a life lesson at the way to assist us expand our cognizance. As everything we revel in allows us extend our interest and increase, the card on this function is of outstanding assist to delve into what we're wearing out. It will lead us to more recognition, no matter whether or not or now not the result is superb or terrible. The card on this function will become what we need to test more carefully.

As has already been clarified, in magic and the occult, the Celtic waft plays an crucial and direct characteristic within the use of Tarot Cards. The Celtic pass characteristic lets in one to visualize future effects and obta n facts on particular questions that one continues in mind. This shape of magic allows us to attain specific possibilities concerning the close to and distant future after which follow particular pointers. In truth, there may be some thing essential that we must recollect: we need to make clean to whom we're throwing the gambling playing cards.

It is set the effect this will have on the character for whom the cardboard analyzing is being finished. With this, we aren't defining their destiny or sealing it however as an alternative indicating what the playing cards display us. The individual accountable for what takes area might be the protagonist, as they'll understand a manner to reply and act concerning what they've got determined out about their future. Magic does now not determine what is going to appear to us; it virtually clarifies the panorama for us. We are people who can trade it and do something positive about it, usually.

Chapter 8: The Ankh or Egyptian Cross

History and use of the Egyptian Cross

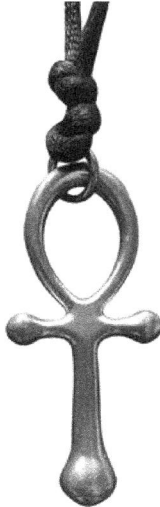

History

Origins of the Egyptian Cross

The Egyptian bypass or the akh is one of the most recognizable symbols of ancient Egypt, referred to as "the important thing of ife" or "the pass of existence." This dates from the Archaic Dynastic Period (c. 3150-2613 BCE). The go is formed by using immediately strains that intersect, collectively with proper angles at the top, that may be a loop or oval with a cope with form. This image is given the which means of lifestyles and grow to be appreciably carried out in historic Egyptian tradition.

Not masses is notion approximately the start location of this photograph from ancient Egypt because it changed proper into a civilization with very mysterious and summary symbols. The pass may be seen in masses of hieroglyphs and representations of vintage Egyptian gods posing with it in hand or on staff. Due to its peculiar shape, it got here to provide different names, which encompass the critical factor to Egypt and the crucial issue to the Nile. It become even called the pass of life. The move is considered a normal signal. The Egyptians called it the ankh, and it changed into considered a mystical key that opened the border to immortality.

Use of the Egyptian Cross

Over the years, the Egyptian pass has been used by specific cultures and for diverse functions, which incorporates as a enchantment for great achievement, as a pendulum for recovery, and to help us find out answers to our questions.

Crosses are ubiquitous and can be located in cultures as wonderful because the Phoenician, Persian, Etruscan, Greek, Scandinavian, Celtic, African, Australian, Chinese,Tibetan, Iroquois, Navajo, Aztec, Mayan, Incan and the Aymaran cultures.

The Egyptian pass or ankh is a effective active picture used as a healing tool. These characteristics of the ankh are identified through the usage of Alama, this is why it's far utilized in severa recovery approaches, having a huge power and a very excessive vibrational frequency whilst connecting with Universal love to apply its homes. Alama remedy turned into superior via the psychologist Valeria Mandakovic in 2010. This remedy can heal symptoms, troubles, and illnesses of a wide variety (emotional, bodily, intellectual, relationships) from the idea. In this strength treatment, the affected person is lively and the protagonist of their recovery. The person is aware what their signs and signs and symptoms and issues are, and it is they who heal themselves, with the therapist's guidance.

The goddess of the pride of life and loss of life (Hathor) gave existence with the flow of ankh, and, in lots of respects, this picture is associated with the goddesses Inanna, Ishtar, Astarte, Aphrodite, and Venus. The Egyptians official the ankh go as a spiritual photo and used it in the path of Egyptian neb-ankh meditation and various healing rituals.

Current practitioners of Egyptian magic maintain to use this picture as a effective energizer and enhancer of their rites and a key to open cosmic electricity. Healers use it to relieve and remedy illnesses and illnesses.

Today, the ankh or Egyptian pass is taken into consideration an energetic talisman, an active amulet, which generates subtle emissions of beneficial radiation, detectable by means of dowsing techniques. It is said to be the most effective talisman noted to mankind. Many people use the Egyptian pass as a manner of divination and as an opportunity remedy to make clear problems, stability the energy of our chakras, and search for misplaced gadgets and missing individuals.

The Egyptian pass may be manufactured from metallic, metal alloys carved into gem stones, crystals, wood, clay, or stone surfaces. Occultists endorse that metal crosses be used as personal amulets, on the identical time as wooden, clay, or stone carvings are higher perfect to the protection of the house. Likewise, an Egyptian pass carved out of a crystal may be an extraordinary talisman of fitness.

If you make a decision to apply the Egyptian pass as a pendulum, you can consecrate it inside the equal way as defined in financial disaster III.

Chapter 9: The Phases of the Moon

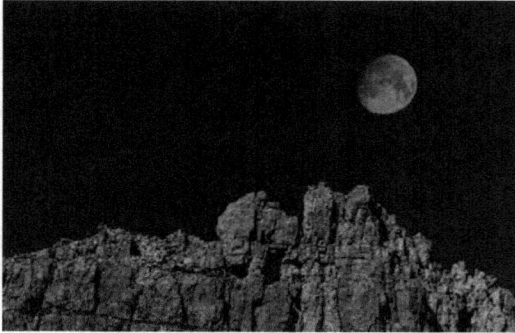

How Do the Lunar Phases Influence Our Life?

The word moon has its beginning in Latin and way "luminous" or "the only that illuminates." The moon is clearly one in every of a number of the mysteries of the universe. It isn't always mentioned for sure how or whilst it came to be. The truth is that the moon had tremendous meanings in unique cultures spherical the arena.

According to the ideals of our ancestors, the moon at once impacts the tides, agriculture, the united states of america of mind in people, animals, and other living beings in all its additives. These beliefs were a legacy that has subsequently been practiced and endured for plenty generations.

Ancient Egyptian hieroglyphs are in which we discover the primary writings wherein the moon's impact on people is described. Before the Egyptians commenced out worshiping the solar because the very best determine, they glorified the moon.

In Western astrology, the moon represents the man or woman's emotional nature, which characterizes the inner infant that everyone deliver inside. In addition, the cult of the moon existed in ancient Greece, Babylon, India, and China, and the Moon performed a essential role in the advent of calendars due to its predictable changes. Many cultures used the positions of the moon to perform magic.

Every month bestows a contemporary opportunity to analyze and mirror on wherein we're and in which we want to move. Knowing every moon phase and all of the houses that every one has makes it less hard to take benefit of all its magic and electricity to reinvent ourselves and begin over. Here you can find the four number one ranges of the moon and a way to use them for your advantage. Get rid of bad behavior, toxic relationships, and terrible energies.

New moon: Better called Black Moon: When we do not see the moon, it is in the famous waning section. The New Moon is an brilliant time to push away all negatives, cleanse your self, or start a healthy eating plan. It isn't certainly useful to create some factor new inside the route of this time.

Crescent moon: This moon section is one of the most terrific levels for the whole thing, together with beginning relationships, a task, or a business employer and regaining power. In magic, we always use this phase to growth and accumulate all our purposes, as an instance, love, coins, health, and fertility. If you want your hair and nails to develop more potent, you have to cut them during this moon segment. Also is an excellent time to carry out any ritual geared toward enhancing your existence.

Full moon: In this segment, the moon is in all its beauty, and it's miles the extraordinary time to acquire all of your dreams. If you have quartz, amulets, valuable stones, and pendulums, it is right to fee them with proper energy. To price them with the moon's magic, you need to place them in your balcony or window all through the night time. The whole moon is favorable for doing rituals inquiring for an high-quality monetary tool. If you need to increase your intuition or your psychic capabilities you may do it inside the path of this moon phase. Meditation and manifesting what you need on a whole moon will help you bought what you want.

Waning moon: During this section, you can supply an stop to relationships, situations, or incomplete topics. In magic, we use this section to lessen the whole lot horrible for us, like complex friendships, poisonous relationships, the evil eye, illness, dependencies, etc., breaking up the terrible energies and removing the entirety that hurts us.

CHAPTER 10: WHAT IS A PENDULUM?

A pendulum is a divination tool this is used to determine the truth based totally on your cutting-edge-day fact. It is likewise steering out of your higher self, your spirit crew, surpassed loved ones, your ancestors, or any spirit which you preference to speak with. It permits to assemble your intuition and your discernment.

Discernment is a totally essential component in navigating your religious adventure, that is why the pendulum is this sort of useful tool.

Pretty a remarkable deal something that can keep from your hand and swing may be used as a pendulum. Necklaces are the most not unusual alternative, however even keys on a lanyard want to work in a pinch.

Then, once you're equipped for a actual pendulum, you should purchase a handmade one at thatsoulglow.Com.

CHAPTER 11: HOW TO PICK THE RIGHT PENDULUM

Picking the right pendulum might be very crucial. Trying to work with a pendulum that is not best on your electricity also car result in unenthusiastic or wrong solutions. The more that you art work with a pendulum, the extra that you could understand that special pendulums have one in every of a type "personalities". Certain pendulums come into your life to art work with you for unique conditions, and aren't that usefu with different areas of your existence. Whereas exclusive pendulums are multi-cause. For example, I actually have a pendulum specially for speakme with my ancestors, one for the times that I am tuning in with my internal toddler, higher self, and shadow self. Once you're cushty with using a pendulum, you may be guided to buy extra.

If you are shopping for a pendulum from a crystal store, you have the benefit of asking it, if it's far the proper pendulum for you.

If you've got used a pendulum earlier than, preserve up the pendulum, and for your head ask, "are you the pendulum for me right now?" and it'll allow you to realise sure or no. Your commands will generally be just like each pendulum you operate. You can double check via asking the pendulum to show you a certain and a no. If you have got were given in no way used a pendulum earlier than, have a look at beforehand to discover ways to software program a pendulum or, you may use your instinct!

Using your instinct to pick out a pendulum:

The more which you use your pendulum, the greater that you may recognize which you don't in reality make errors. There is continuously a cause why you do the belongings you do. Trust your self, and pick out the first pendulum which you were interested in. Then, in a while, appearance up the recuperation houses of the crystal linked in your pendulum. If you obtain a wooden or steel pendulum, look up the houses of wood/metal pendulums. You are going to be validated precisely why you picked an appropriate pendulum for you. And much like that, you have built a chunk more self guarantee for your intuitive competencies.

If you are buying your pendulum online you will basically do the equal steps as above, however in preference to the use of a pendulum which you manifestly do not have, you'll use a necklace or a lanyard to invite. OR you may use your intuition to choose.

CHAPTER 12: HOW TO CLEANSE A PENDULUM

The first issue which you want to do while you get a brand new pendulum, is cleanse it. Regularly cleaning your pendulum is what is going to make the distinction, from your pendulum lasting for weeks vs. Years. Cleansing it additionally guarantees which you are best operating at the facet of your private strength, and not every body who has touched the pendulum in advance than you acquire it.

Smoke Cleansing:

You can smoke cleanse a pendulum using sage, palo santo, mugwort, incense, and so forth. Simply preserve the pendulum over the smoke. The pendulum will normally pass in a circle and save you spinning as soon as it's far cleansed. The more that it spins, the more energy it had on it.

Cleansing with Selenite:

You can cleanse your pendulum via setting it on a chunk of selenite or in a selenite bowl.

This method generally first-class calls for a few minutes.

Sound Cleansing:

If you have got a tuning fork or a valid bowl, you can use sound frequency to cleanse your pendulum. Simply play the frequency and hover it throughout the pendulum.

How to recognise at the same time as a pendulum wants to be cleansed:

The easiest way to apprehend if a pendulum wants to be cleansed, is by way of asking it. Or you can appearance out for the subsequent signs.

Signs that your pendulum needs to be cleansed:

● Your pendulum swings start getting small.

● Your pendulum is non-responsive.

● Your pendulum chain receives tangled.

● Your pendulum maintains falling.

● Your pendulum starts feeling heavier.

- You get a experience that your pendulum wishes to be cleansed. (That's your instinct.)

Pendulums absorb electricity, a few quicker than others. If you are round masses of human beings on a each day foundation, your pendulum will want to be cleansed greater often. Before you permit all of us touch your pendulum, ask your pendulum "is it ok if I permit _____ touch/use you?"

If a pendulum is going too prolonged with out being cleansed, it will damage.

If a pendulum breaks, use a necklace or a lanyard and ask:

1. Did my pendulum spoil because it needed to be cleansed?

2. Should I located the pendulum lower again collectively?

three. Did my pendulum ruin because it fulfilled its reason?

four. Does the pendulum need me to keep any a part of it?

5. Does the pendulum need to be disposed or want to I burry it?

CHAPTER 13: HOW TO PROGRAM A PENDULUM

Always ask questions about your head to avoid trickster strength influencing your solutions. Hold your pendulum but you enjoy maximum comfortable, virtually make sure you keep it from the pinnacle, and supply it room to swing. Shaky fingers do not rely, you could though get accurate solutions. You can use your pendulum in a transferring automobile, or maybe closer to strong wind, and the solutions will even though be correct.

It's essential to utility your pendulum to only acquire answers out of your higher self till you channel a selected spirit.

To do that, say: "I claim that every one pendulums that I use now, or will use inside the future, will incredible deliver me answers that come from my better self till I in particular country in any other case." While saying this your pendulum may also additionally bypass in circles or vibrate a chunk in your hand, which means the pendulum is responding for your electricity.

If a pendulum does no longer respond on the same time as programming, try carrying it with you, and sound asleep with it for your pillowcase for 3 days and 3 nights, to permit it to connect to your energy. If it's going to in spite of the reality that no longer respond to your strength, strive the use of some other pendulum, or a necklace. As I mentioned earlier, the use of the right pendulum on the identical time as you're dealing with powerful strength makes all the difference.

Now, we will get into programming your hints in your pendulum. After you assert a command, you may civilly (sure with courtesy, it makes a distinction) inform your pendulum to save you shifting. This goes to show you the magic of your pendulum and also help you distinguish the guidelines.

Programming instructions:

While preserving up your pendulum say:

"display me a sure."

"please prevent"

"show me a no."

"please prevent"

"show me what it looks as if after I am asking something that I can not apprehend the answer to." (Your pendulum may be actually despite the fact that for this one, this is ok!)

"please prevent"

"Show me what it seems like even as trickster energy is spherical."

All of those guidelines are very important to installation together along with your pendulum so please do not bypass any. If the commands that your pendulum gives you are difficult, you can utility your pendulum to move inside the path that you would like it to move in. For instance, if you would like your sure swings to be up and down you virtually ask your pendulum to make the sure direction up and down.

There are some subjects that we can't recognize the answer to. If you do no longer have the direction installation that helps you to comprehend that you're asking approximately a few issue which you cannot recognize approximately, you could be wondering it's far offering you with a solution even as it's far in reality in search of to offer you a sign that it can not solution your query.

Some examples of factors which you can not ask your pendulum:

• Questions approximately whilst you or a person else is going to bypass away.

• Questions about others that do not have any correlation to you. That manner nope, you can't ask about Barbra's cheating boyfriend, till Barbra desires you to ask your pendulum approximately her boyfriend.

• Gambling. Oh what a global it is probably if we have to get the lotto numbers with a pendulum! Unfortunately, except you are destined to claim your abundance through the lottery or the jackpot in a on line casino, you may not have lots genuine fortune using a pendulum for playing. However, if it's far your fate to claim your wealth in that manner, (all you have to do is ask your pendulum) then thru all method, play away!

Tread gently with being pregnant questions.

At the give up of the day keep in mind, your pendulum will assist you to realise even as you are asking a question that you cannot realise the solution to as long as you've got were given that path set up.

Sometimes if you have very huge moments in your life, or you have a large mindset shift, the route of your pendulum swings may additionally additionally exchange. The pendulum has its personal way of telling you that the pointers have changed.

How to apprehend if your instructions have changed:

If your solutions start getting perplexing, that may be a most important signal that your commands have switched. To check, keep up your pendulum and say "show me a sure". If the swing is opposite than what you had it programmed for, it switched. Simply reprogram your pendulum with your chosen suggestions.

How to deal with trickster energy:

If you get alerted that there's a trickster spirit spherical you, get rid of it through manner of asking your ancestors, spirit team, the Universe, God, whomever you work with to cast off the trickster power. Say: "_____ please do away with the trickster power from my area". Your pendulum must bypass in a circle till the strength is lengthy gone. The more potent the electricity, the longer it will preserve spinning. If you cannot dispose of the trickster energy strive cleansing your pendulum and your vicinity. Then, decide out in which the trickster strength came from. We will communicate more on pinpointing the start of negative strength in monetary wreck 6.

CHAPTER 14: HOW TO BUILD TRUST WITH YOUR PENDULUM

Be prepared for the journey of a lifetime at the same time as constructing don't forget with your higher self. Your higher self doesn't see things as black and white like we do. Your better self is balanced, and may see the bigger picture in each state of affairs which you go through. So at the same time as asking for steerage out of your higher self, absolutely understand that it's miles going to be what is on your maximum actual. What's to your maximum particular isn't always comfortable, or may not appear the maximum logical...However it constantly works out. If you can learn how to see the larger photo genuinely as your higher self does, you can thrive.

Example: One time I modified into searching for to determine out what store I should get canine food from. My pendulum grow to be telling me that I shouldn't go to the shop that I first off had planned. My husband was already on the manner to the real keep and we were surely approximately to go out, however I actually have end up telling him the pendulum knowledgeable me no. He insisted that we flow because of the fact we had been right there. So we pass internal, and I sense all of this power spherical me. I were given the chills and couldn't stop shaking on the identical time as in the shop. They had an event going on that day, and I modified into selecting up the electricity from all of the people there. They didn't actually have the food that we had been searching out!

So every so often the steerage out of your better self might not seem to make experience in a logical way, but the large picture makes feel. The massive photograph is that even though I ended up going someplace that I "wasn't supposed to cross", I received information via that revel in. I gained the know-how of understanding that my pendulum has my exceptional interest, and that I want to be aware of it. I absolutely have seen people learn to be privy to their pendulum in harsher strategies so I am glad that I placed with the sort of small scenario. Hopefully you can test from that small example that I went thru as nicely, so that you don't want to go through a tough scenario to recognize that you want to continuously concentrate for your pendulum.

Do not ask for steering on a subject except you are prepared to confront each final results. Do now not attempt to make the pendulum alternate its answer. It will normally sincerely change its solution, to let you undergo a situation as a manner to show you why it gave you the unique answer.

You can manipulate the pendulum collectively in conjunction with your mind, however you realize the difference among asking and telling. Ask your query, don't overthink it. Let the solution go with the flow through your frame, on your pendulum. You are the device. You already have all the answers you are searching for, receive as actual with your self. That is basically what you are doing, constructing trust inner your self.

Start with little alternatives. Anytime you want to make a small desire, like which grocery maintain to visit, which meals to eat for dinner, or perhaps which direction to take home. Let your pendulum make those selections for you. Things that wouldn't certainly have massive effects. Like I said in advance than, it isn't normally the maximum logical aspect that our pendulums tel us to do. Sometimes there's a bigger reason. So your pendulum can also additionally allow you to recognize to take the longer path home but perhaps it's miles so you can keep away from an unsightly twist of destiny, or likely you be conscious a few difficulty that conjures up your advertising method, or you become walking into a person which you haven't seen in a surely long term. The pendulum/your higher self has a motive for telling you the topics that it tells you.

On our spiritual journey masses of factors regularly don't make feel till we get to a positive factor in our course, wherein we are able to see the scenario objectively. That is in which we find peace.

Using Tarot To Strengthen Your Trust With A Pendulum:

Another top notch way to build your instinct and assemble your do not forget collectively along with your pendulum is to apply pick-a-card readings on YouTube. This will beef up your instinct and your belief in different varieties of divination as nicely.

To get began observe those steps:

1. Look for a pick out-a-card analyzing that peaks your interest.

2. Let your pendulum determine the only that you need to take a look at.

3. Pick the pile(s) intuitively. What does your instinct say is the right pile(s) for you?

four. Use your pendulum to see which pile(s) you have been purported to pick. Was it the identical pile(s) your intuition picked?

5. Watch the choose out-a-card video and notice if it resonates.

Let the pendulum take the wheel:

The final way to construct your believe together along with your pendulum is to completely give up. As you go through your religious journey you may find out that surrendering is the vital component to peace. Surrender manage.

Pick a day that you will permit your pendulum make all the alternatives for you. Every. Single. Decision. This is going to spotlight some subjects on your existence that perhaps you aren't being attentive to. Why might your pendulum can help you recognize now not to reply to someone's text?Why would not it allow you to understand to preserve at a terrific grocery keep?

You can have a look at masses about yourself on the same time as doing this exercising, and it's far a amusing way to assemble your accept as actual with along with your pendulum.

CHAPTER 15: GETTING TO THE ROOT OF NEGATIVE ENERGY

You need to cast off any outdoor influences that would lead you down an prolonged and further difficult path for your manifestations.

Some people need to dismiss terrible power. They sense that inside the occasion that they don't do not forget in it, then it doesn't exist. But you want to be real with your self and recognize that during any truth there can be going to be horrible electricity. You cannot change that irrespective of what number of timelines you bounce into, but what you could do is transmute that terrible energy. But first, you have to recognize that it's even there. You have in order to come to be aware about what's coming from you, and what is an out of doors have an impact on. This goes to be the aspect wherein you begin to unlearn the programming which have emerge as programmed inside you, and honestly start to find out who you truely are.

A lot of the time we don't even understand that the power that we are feeling, the emotions that we deliver, the way that we react, is honestly coming from terrible energy influencing us. Trickster energy or lousy electricity. This electricity served a reason proper now, however we have had been given now reached the point in which we do not want this form of strength influencing our frequency anymore.

To get to the basis of lousy power, use your pendulum to ask yourself those questions:

● Ask your self in which the electricity got here from and notice if the answer pops into your head. Confirm on the side of your pendulum.

● Ask if the electricity came from an outside source.

● Ask if the strength came from an emotion which you were feeling.

● Ask if the energy got here from something past this realm. (if you're willing to transport down that rabbit hollow)

With asking these questions you want to be capable of slender down in which the strength got here from.

Now ask your pendulum if there may be a few element which you are alleged to do with this information. If it tells you no, then carry on. If it says positive, then ask those questions:

• Do you want me to investigate a few aspect from this enjoy?

• Was this revel in meant to expose up?

• Ask your steerage group to deliver you signs and symptoms and symptoms and signs about what the larger image is from this situation.

When identifying in which the awful energy got here from it's now not due to the fact you need to deliver horrific strength decrease back, it's miles because you want to be privy to what is going on spherical you. There is usually a lesson in the good buy that you undergo. People are not clearly attacking you with lousy energy, there's constantly a bigger photo.

Addressing your council

What approximately while the terrible power isn't coming from an outdoor supply? What if it's your internal critic? We will call the critic or critic(s), your council.

You are not helpless to this critic and you will be amazed to research that it isn't always you the least bit.

Ask your self this query: Who runs my inner council? See who comes up on your mind, and then see in case your pendulum confirms it. Usually it is a person who raised you or has/had loads of have an effect on on you. If it is one in each of your dad and mom, it's far the spirit of them, they might however be alive and be strolling your council. We are multidimensional beings. Our spirit bodies can be in lots of locations right now, the ones human beings do no longer consciously realize that they'll be on foot your council.

Once you choose out who is running your council, ask your pendulum in case you want to get rid of that man or woman from your council.

If it says to dispose of them, keep your pendulum and say "I take away _____ from my council" and ensure to characteristic in something about why you enjoy like it is time to put off that man or woman out of your council. This is in which a piece of shadow work is to be had in. These humans served a reason in walking our council, they have been given us to this very component in our lifestyles. Be grateful for at least that.

When putting off a member from your council, the pendulum will make a circle till the character has been eliminated. The longer that the pendulum spins, the more of a power they likely had over your existence.

If your pendulum says that the character does now not need to be removed, however it is a person apart from you, it is able to not be time to get rid of them out of your council right now. This can also need to trade later.

Sometimes council individuals aren't recognized as human beings; they'll be diagnosed as character traits.

Example: If you are continuously going through concept loops in which you are experiencing jealous behavior, then ask your pendulum if there may be any individual on your council this is jealous. If it says high-quality, remove them. After putting off a member you will possibly sense a shift on your frame and in a while a shift to your attitude. Sometimes you may be confirmed the areas on your lifestyles in which the problem started otherwise you might be proven techniques to combat the issue.

This is a awesome way to do shadow art work and it's an incredible manner to get to the idea of terrible self speak.

CHAPTER 16: CHECKING YOUR CHAKRAS WITH A PENDULUM

When we've got unaligned chakras it affects plenty in our lifestyles and plenty on our spiritual journey. We frequently have a study the zero.33 eye and proper away try to open it, but what approximately the alternative six chakras? We have seven chakras that are associated with our bodily frame. Each of the chakras do a little factor superb and play an vital feature inside the subjects which may be taking place in our existence.

Let's communicate approximately the incredible meanings of the chakras, so that you can see how crucial it's far to have your chakras aligned.

The root chakra has to do collectively together along with your balance and feeling steady. Located at the bottom of your backbone. It is related to the colours: red, brown, and black. An unaligned root chakra can reason feelings of worry, anxiety, lack mentality, or a whole brush aside for your safety.

The sacral chakra has to do together along with your sexuality and your creativity. Located under your stomach button. It is associated with the colour orange. An unaligned sacral chakra can reason hypersexuality, feeling uninspired, or loss of creativity.

The solar plexus chakra has to do with yourself belief and your happiness. Located below your ribs. It is associated with the coloration yellow. An unaligned solar plexus can motive emotions of despair, low self-worth, or a superiority complex.

The coronary heart chakra has to do at the side of your potential to offer and acquire love. Located at the center of your chest. It is associated with inexperienced and red. Someone with an unaligned coronary heart chakra is closed off to love, unaffectionate, or too loving to folks which might be unworthy.

The throat chakra has to do togethe‍ with your capacity to talk authentically. Located at your throat. It is related to blue and slight blue. An unaligned throat chakra shows up by means of manner of lying, gossiping, or now not speakme up for yourself.

The 1/3 eye chakra has to do on the aspect of your ability to appearance what can not be visible in conjunction with your physical eyes. Located in among your eyebrows. It is associated with indigo blue and crimson. An unaligned 1/three eye chakra effects in being unimaginative, feeling stuck, loss of clarity, or strolling wild together at the side of your creativeness (going overboard).

The crown chakra is your potential to hook up with your better self, spirit and the divine. Located at the pinnacle of your head. It is related to the colours: white, gold, and red. A person with an unaligned crown chakra can be closed off to divine reviews, or very withdrawn from human connections.

You can use your pendulum to check for chakra imbalances truly via soaring your pendulum in the front of every chakra.

Here is how you'll direct your pendulum:

-If the chakra is open, swing in the course that my body is dealing with. (up and down)

-If the chakra is closed, then swing inside the course opposite of the manner that my frame is dealing with. (aspect to facet)

Go via every chakra and look at which ones are blocked and which of them are open. This can trade indoors a right away so just understand that it's far great a image of your modern electricity. This does not imply that a chakra is generally going to be closed, nor does it mean that a chakra is continuously going to be open.

There are numerous wearing events that you could do to open and stability every chakra. When you have got a look at that a chakra isn't balanced, say "how is my _____ chakra so balanced?" When you located your affirmation in the form of a question it makes your brain cross searching out the answer. Just like each time you spot a certain form of car one time and then all of a shocking you begin seeing it over and over yet again. Your brain does that for many stuff, and you could software your mind for what you wart it to do. Set the goal and watch what comes your way. Once you begin getting the ones thoughts or as I like to call them, downloads, you may ask your pendulum if this positive concept is some detail that you want to pursue to stability your chakra.

The solution want to come to you fast, or it would even come to you subconsciously. You can also furthermore start doing subjects that you don't even realise are without a doubt supposed to align that chakra. That is the lovable element approximately programming ourselves and putting intentions, our unconscious absolutely takes over. Your instinct is privy to exactly wherein to guide you. You truly need to consider yourself.

CHAPTER 17: YOUR PHYSICAL HEALTH

It's vital to word that unbalanced chakras can result in bodily illnesses or illnesses. Think of, as above, so under. A lot of the topics that people undergo, need to do with very unbalanced or closed chakras.

That's why it's essential to heal!

If inside the course of your journey you begin to feel a few component that feels out of the regular, ask your pendulum if it has some issue to do with any of your chakras, it can be an enhance to that chakra.

Your pendulum isn't always going to make you forget about about your health. If you need medical interest, your pendulum will will let you realize to visit the medical medical doctor. Our higher self can be very plenty in pick people getting medical hobby at the same time as we want it.

Medication

Some humans surely want medicine. It's important to determine out what works exquisite for you. If you are presently taking remedy and are unsure in case you need to hold taking it or not, ask your better self for steering. It's no longer going to make you stop taking your treatment if this is some issue that is on your best hobby.

Connecting on your frame.

Once you connect with your body, you recognize how

powerful your frame can be! Start with the aid of asking your frame what it likes and what it doesn't like.

Here's some questions you can ask your frame to get you started out:

- Does my frame like dairy?

- Does my body like meat?

- Does my body want to stick to a specific food plan?

- Does my body much like the water that I drink?

- Does my frame like soda?

- Does my frame now not like certain additives that I currently eat? (bear in mind substances that make your stomach upset, or cause you to break out, and so forth.)

You can redesign your body in reality by way of honoring what it likes. Programming Your Body

Now which you understand what your body likes and what your frame doesn't like, you may tell your body the way you need it to keep the meals which you eat. Be very particular. Think approximately how you would really like your body to keep your fat. Do you need it to keep extra fats for your hips or your thighs, and so on. Maybe you want your fat to be transmuted into muscle. Once you decide, hold up your pendulum and inform your body in which you want it to store your fat. Then say, "frame, you're to put off any extra fat through_____"(peeing, pooping, or sweating). The desire is as much as you, however ensure which you're particular on how you want your body to eliminate excess fats, or it'll pick for you. Your pendulum should flow in a circle while you're setting those intentions and it will forestall as soon as the intentions are set.

Then, inform your body which you would love for it to "transmute all toxins into vitamins, and get rid of any excess nutrients via _____", in something way you decide.

The manner that meals transmutation manifests bodily is super! Intuitively, you will know what to gravitate towards to make your food transmutation process the easiest.

When you're transmuting electricity, you want to be precise on wherein you have become this power from. If you aren't particular approximately in which you get the strength from you'll be the usage of your personal power, and it could depart you exhausted. Set your aim by means of pronouncing, "I set the aim that each one power that I transmute, comes from the universe's existence force electricity". The universe has an endless amount of strength and it is a really perfect area to drag from so you can keep yours.

CHAPTER 18: SHADOW WORK

Shadow paintings is the process of addressing the elements of you which you try and disguise from others and deny about your self. But much like a shadow, this stuff are usually around. The global is continually mirroring these items to you. It's hidden in your triggers. Shadow work gives you the opportunity to learn how to perceive the shadow/ego, and integrate it along with your better self. To start shadow work, take a look at your thoughts and triggers.

Working via triggers

When you get induced through some thing, ask your pendulum the subsequent questions:

● Is my higher self dissatisfied about this?

● Is my ego dissatisfied about this?

● Is my inner infant disillusioned about this?

● Should I stay dissatisfied?

Getting the answer to these questions is going to offer you a few angle on why to procure brought about. For example if it changed into your internal toddler, perhaps the issue that brought about you changed into which you had been dealt with that way whilst you had been a toddler.

Now which you figured out what it's miles that honestly made you disillusioned, you have to permit pass. Give gratitude for the instant, due to the fact the bigger image is that it highlighted the shadow work that you needed to deal with.

Shadow work is the fastest manner to transport ahead on your adventure.

Break out of these cycles.

Lastly recall, shadow paintings will show up while it wishes to be confronted, you do not need to head searching out it.

CHAPTER 19: DECODING SYNCHRONICITIES

Everything is divine and in case you take the time to ask your pendulum, you could parent out what nearly the entirety way on your life. We marvel a lot but we do no longer need to be left wondering...

Using the net to determine out what synchronicities imply for you:

1. If it is an angel number, an animal, a image, a shade, etc. Search at the internet for "the non secular that means of _____."

2. Use your pendulum to figure out which website is the one that has the which means in it for you.

The meanings of synchronicities are going to be exceptional for each person. It all depends on what you as an character pay attention to. A individual might see a variety of numbers, colors, symbols, listen different sounds, smell unique smells, and so forth. And that is how their spirit crew will communicate to them.

You also can ask your pendulum the following questions:

- Is this sign a message from a handed loved one?

- Is this signal a message from my spirit guide(s)?

- Is this signal a message from (the Universe, God, Source, angels, and so forth.)

- Is this sign a message for me to be careful?

- Is this sign to reveal me that I am cherished?

- Is this a sign to expose me that I am protected?

- Should I look more into this signal?

CHAPTER 20: INTEGRATION - USING YOUR BODY AS A PENDULUM

Our our bodies clearly respond to reality. Hence the invention of lie detector assessments.

Using your body as a pendulum is referred to as body checking out. To body take a look at, you're taking the identical steps as you did with your pendulum. Ask it to show you a sure, no, and an I don't need to know. Observe what happens for your body and what you experience, see, or pay attention when you ask about every answer. Maybe a yes looks like a tugging in your stomach, or for a no, you hear an aircraft sound on your head.

Eventually you're going to paintings up to the point where you best need a pendulum to confirm matters that seem wild past your creativeness. For the whole thing else you'll learn how to use your frame to navigate your decisions. This is the ultimate level up in terms of discernment; that is when you actually recognise that you are the device.

There's a lot facts accessible! The primary device that you may have on your journey is discernment. Now which you have all this expertise, you may live to tell the tale, and thrive for your spiritual adventure. Be intentional and enforce using your pendulum each day. I wish you're excited because your lifestyles is set to trade.

Chapter 21: Meet the Pendulum

What Is a Pendulum?

A pendulum is a weight suspended via a string or a series and allowed to swing backward and forward freely. They come in many unique sizes and styles, but all of them have one issue in not unusual – they appearance actually, actually cool. Originally, they were used to expose the motion of the heavens.

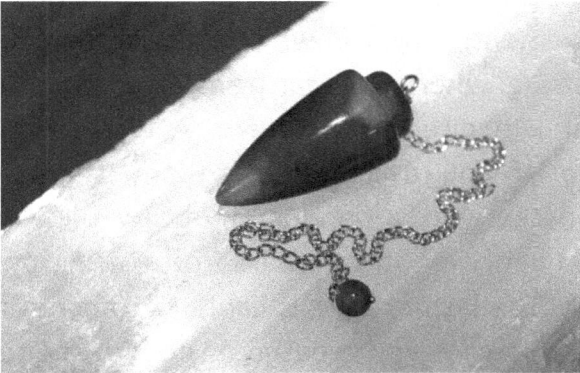

Scientists and feature studied the mechanics in the returned of pendulums for masses of years. In quite simple terms, the principle concept is that, because it travels, power passes through a space-time continuum. As energy actions from one vicinity to some other, the gap the various 2 points is distorted, and this distortion creates anxiety in time and area. As such, strength will take the shortest and least resisting route via this vicinity-time continuum, because of this that energy flows from in which it originates to where it's going.

Pendulums characteristic on this number one principle of strength go with the flow. When you place a pendulum in a rustic of movement, power flows down thru the chain or string, wherein it's far transferred anyplace your aim directs it to head. A word to the wise: If you're going to do any shape of divination with a pendulum, opt for one with a sequence or string in area of a string on a stick. The latter range is liable to transferring round in case you breathe or possibly twitch, in the end they may be predisposed to be less correct.

This exercise is much like what is known as dowsing (a divination technique to find out radiations from all the subjects round us), but the difference is that this method makes use of a pendulum in choice to a dowsing rod. In this case, you have a piece of string or chain with a bit at the bottom. You maintain immediately to at the least one prevent and swing it in the front of someone else, asking questions about what you're seeking out out about. If you shake it up and down for "certain" then thing to side for "no," that gives you your answer. The pendu um is commonly used for topics like love, health, career, charge range, and extra.

History of Pendulum Magic

Many ancient cultures have used pendulums to foresee the destiny because of the reality that point immemorial. For example, in Chinese fortune telling, a pendulum is regularly held over the pinnacle of a new child toddler to inform if they may be blessed with accurate health and wealth. In Europe, early authorities inside the occult movement would grasp crystals above their beds at night time to guard them from evil spirits.

In Western subculture, pendulums have constantly been used as a way of fortune-telling. A famous approach to are watching for the destiny includes using pendulum gizmos or wind-up toys that make a swinging noise while shaken and a clicking noise at the same time as they come to relaxation. These gizmos had been utilized by fortune-teller in historical Egypt, Greece, and Rome to test out the destiny. In Ancient Egypt, adepts have to shake a crystal putting from their neck, and if it made a clicking noise, it meant specific fitness for fifty years and non violent nights of sleep. However, if the press noise have become placed through a thumping noise it intended lousy success for fifty years.

How to Choose Your Pendulum

How do you pick out a pendulum for pendulum magic? What should you endure in thoughts at the same time as seeking out the right one on your practice? As a guiding principle, you need to don't forget the fabric it's made from. When looking for pendulums, there are separate attributes you want to preserve in thoughts: substances and developments.

Materials

Materials can be separated into instructions — steel and plastic. The most famous materials humans use within the West are brass and copper. Plastic is a extra current advent to pendulum use however has examined to be fairly effective as wel. The most commonplace sort of plastic used is acrylic. Both brass and copper had been used to create all varieties of equipment inside the path of records, which encompass the axe, spear, and arrowhead. They have proven themselves time and time another time as the exceptional desire for pendulum use.

When I begin looking at substances, I check the neck of the device. Essentially, the neck is what determines how lengthy the fabric will final earlier than it wears out. Choosing a neck that's too long technique your pendulum will now not be able to carry out any magic rapid. Choose an prolonged neck in case you expect the usage of it for a while and want it to closing longer. Longer necks are simpler to grip. By contrast, choosing a short neck approach your pendulum also can feel heavier and much a good deal less responsive on your hand. Choosing a tall, slender neck will increase the rate at which it may spin. Choose a light-weight fabric to make it extra correct, while a strong fabric can increase the texture

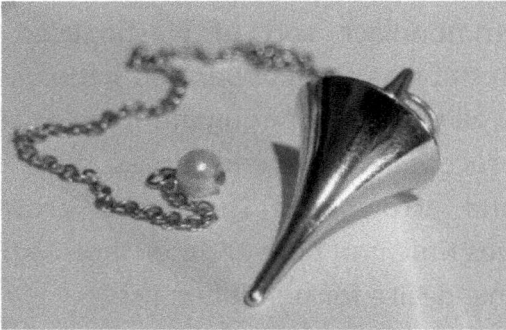

of manage you have were given at the same time as the use of it.

Brass is by using far atop my listing of preferred materials to apply due to its durability and price-effectiveness. Quartz crystal pendulums are generally not as durable as brass (notwithstanding the reality that they will be superior in a few strategies). They moreover have a tendency to be lots extra costly. Another detail to hold in thoughts is how lengthy your pendulum will final earlier than its effectiveness wears out. If you need to buy one if you need to final a few years, then pick out out a brass pendulum due to the fact it's far the maximum long lasting cloth. While it's going to live on some years without present process any harm, a brass pendulum received't be as durable as a plastic one. At this issue, you need to allow your private preference determine what fabric you pick out.

Characteristics

While seeking out pendulums, recall the developments you need your pendulum to have, as properly. Some attributes that come to thoughts are weight, form, duration, diameter, and loop. The most vital detail to keep in thoughts is they want if you want to spin freely without any friction or play.

A brass pendulum will typically have its weight stamped at the neck of the device, in grains or in kilograms. The not unusual brass pendulum weighs approximately 5-10 grains, but it is able to be heavier or lighter relying for your options. On the simplest hand, a heavier pendulum is much less complicated to govern at the same time as you're transferring it spherical, however it could placed on out faster due to the introduced strain. On the other hand, a lighter pendulum is plenty lots less accurate and greater tough to control for a few human beings, but it wears out slower because of the reduced stress located upon it. For a newbie, I advise beginning with a heavier pendulum until you get used to the way it simply works, and then in all likelihood switching to a lighter one.

A pendulum is fashioned like a flattened cone with the lowest of the cone reduce away to make room for the load. The pendulum's length may be everywhere from 5-30 cm. The extra you put together your axiom, the more important it's miles to pick out out a pendulum that acquired't interfere with its motion. If you are developing a circle of energy, it could be difficult to make adjustments and attain effective elements of your ritual at the identical time as preserving accuracy — in this case, choose out an prolonged pendulum as a substitute.

Dimensions

The diameter is commonly 10-25 mm. If you're developing a circle of energy, it can be difficult to make changes and achieve superb factors of your ritual on the same time as preserving accuracy – in this case, pick a thinner pendulum instead.

The form of the cease will affect how nicely it performs magic. If you need your perdulum to continually thing in the direction of the north (or south, or east, or west), then select out one with a pointed tip. A rounded tip can be used for plenty varieties of magic and doesn't restrict your ritual set-up alternatives as tons. For instance, a flat tip may be used to make a pentacle with a length of string or as an altarpiece. Pendulums with rounded guidelines are the remarkable desire for working magic.

Pendulum lengths range from five-30cm. I in my opinion move for a 20cm pendulum because it's far proper for my pinnacle and hand length. Now, in case you are working with a miles wider circle of strength (say 10-20cm), then a shorter pendulum may fit better for you. If you're on foot with a smaller circle of strength (say five-10cm), pick out out an extended pendulum. Regardless of the dimensions, it is vital to pick out out one that you are cushty with.

As stated, the burden is stamped at the neck of your pendulum in grains or kilograms. Opting each unit of size will mainly rely on your possibilities – each receives the undertaking finished flawlessly. I advise selecting a model amongst 21 grains and 25 grams for novices. This will come up with an concept of the way a pendulum plays while not having to spend more money. If you discover that a particular weight suits your magic and options higher than the opportunity, pick out a heavier or lighter pendulum based totally completely mostly on the way it feels whilst it's far walking magic.

Pendulums are usually made with a loop of string associated with the lowest (like a key chain). Be sure to take away the loop as speedy as you get your new pendulum due to the fact it can be risky if left on at the same time as the usage of it for ritual. The loop of string makes it difficult to perform some forms of rituals as well. It is probably a lot less complex to adjust and reap sure components of your ritual vicinity even as not having to restoration the place of your wrist each time. Make notable not to tie knots within the string because of the truth the pointers of your palms gets caught in it, which may be painful and motive finger damage. A robust knot is useful at the equal time as making an altarpiece or a pentacle, but otherwise, it ought to be eliminated out of your pendulum.

A Few Helpful Tips

If you would love to carry out magic with some one of a kind person, you can want to recollect getting pendulums so each of you may maintain up with the pace. I don't propose using pendulums at once unless you're appearing magic with every different person, as it could get complicated in case you circulate too rapid. If you pick out cut out to apply pendulums, I endorse deciding on ones that have one-of-a-kind substances and characteristics. If the pendulums move too fast whilst you're operating magic, attempt which includes greater strain or slowing down your actions for you to maintain up – this received't normally be viable, but it's nicely properly worth a shot.

For any ritual, it is vital to choose the right weight and length of your pendulum earlier than the usage of it. The purpose is it could be difficult to alter your rituals even as the usage of a pendulum that is each too heavy or too mild. A heavier pendulum may additionally cause greater stress to your hand, which may be tiring whilst using it for lengthy durations of time. If you're simply starting out with magic, choose a lighter pendulum due to the fact it could be much less tough to govern and examine from.

Chapter 22: Making and Working with Your Pendulum

Crafting Your Pendulum

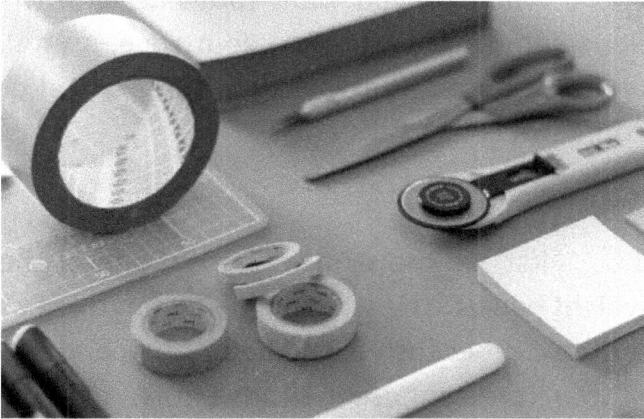

How can you are making your very very own pendulum for magic? The extra hard and personal your pendulum is, the more powerful and powerful it'll be. This manner, it can furthermore emerge as a loved possession for years yet to come.

To make one, you need the following devices:

- A lengthy piece of string or yarn.

- A weight that has been lessen in 1/2 and then drilled or taped in order that it could be hung from the string (non-compulsory).

- An item you want to divine with the pendulum (this is usually a gemstone, crystal, photo of an entity together with an angel or god, tarot card, and so on.).

Instructions:

1. First, tie the string spherical one of the weight halves. The weight may be anything as prolonged because it has been reduce in 1/2 of of. You can use beads, nuts, or little stones.

2. Drill a hole thru it and located a piece of string via the hole (this should be performed in advance than you divide the weight).

3. You also can honestly tie a few string spherical it after which tie the opportunity stop to a comparable-sized bead. However, if you choose to try this and later want to apply this pendulum with some different item which incorporates an Angel card, crystal,

otherwise, you'll each have to update the bead with the item or make your very non-public pendulum from scratch the use of this new object.

Tips: You also can use beads as opposed to one weight. Homeopathic treatments, gemstones, and crystals make correct pendulum weight substitutes. You can area the object within the middle of the string length and tie the ends collectively to form a loop.

Another Way to Make a Pendulum

1.   Grab some string or ribbon and tie it securely at one give up to form a loop about 10cm lengthy. Tie this loop throughout the middle of each one of a kind length of string or ribbon so it forms an L-form. Tie the shorter piece of string to a strong hook, then loop the prolonged piece of string thru this hook. If you need, you could use a key with a hole in it instead of a hook.

2.   Take your prolonged piece of string and tie it around your wrist. Wrap the short piece of string spherical this, so it forms a loop and

sits below your arm. Invert the two portions just so one stop sits on pinnacle of your thumb, after which close to it in so you can maintain it there securely.

3.   You can take a few more string or ribbon to alternate matters up and wrap this loosely round your palm until it forms what seems like a free spiral. Tie it in region with an overhand knot (just like the ones used for tying shoelaces). Then, tie the opportunity surrender to the second one period of string or ribbon and hold close it close to you.

four.   Now, whilst you pass your hand in the the front of you, the pendulum will swing regularly back and forth. The pendulum should prevent swinging at the same time as you maintain your hands despite the reality that (an smooth way to check whether or not or not the device is operating nicely). You also can use your hand as a platform with the resource of extending one finger and touching the string with the alternative.

You now have a pendulum that sways backward and forward on your hand. So, how can this emerge as beneficial for magic?

Alone, or with Friends?

When you eventually have your pendulum, it's splendid to start the use of it on your very own. You don't want to apply it with folks who don't don't forget in what you're doing so it doesn't select up at the strength in their disbelief and skew your results. If you should use it with one-of-a-type human beings, make certain they've got the identical undergo in mind inside the electricity of magic. It sincerely is in your remarkable pursuits to start off to your non-public, so that you can reputation and get better at the usage of your pendulum. As your self perception grows, you could start to show off your skills to others who're truly as interested in pendulum magic as you are.

Which Hand Should You Use?

Although I propose you operate your pendulum at the side of your dominant hand, it couldn't damage to strive using the alternative hand as well whilst you turn out to be gifted with the dominant one. You may additionally look at interesting consequences with the useful resource of switching fingers. When you're working with the pendulum, it's extraordinary as a manner to be sitting so

that you don't sense pressure that would effect the motion of the pendulum.

Sitting or Standing?

Hold on to the pendulum's chain the usage of your forefinger and thumb, and attempt not to maintain it too loosely or tightly. You'll want a table to rest your elbow on so you can be as snug as viable and your body doesn't have an impact at the way the pendulum sways. Note that no unique part of your frame want to the touch the table aside from your elbow, and you need to have your palm going via the floor. Let your pendulum preserve in the front of you. For some human beings, it's simpler to face while the usage of the pendulum. If this is your case, bend your elbow at 90 ranges so it turns into an awful lot much less difficult to hold the pendulum from moving round inconsistently. If you're sitting down, place each toes collectively or pass them on the ankles, which have to slow your pendulum right right down to a save you.

Playing with Length

Now which you have the pendulum placing steady, intentionally swing it, so it actions to and fro. Watch it because it actions in a few thing commands it desires to, and every so often, take control and circulate it in circles as gently as you can. Repeat this motion as you alter the duration of the chain or wire to appearance what period is proper in your pendulum to be greater responsive. A top rule of thumb is to offer it about 5 inches or so (10-15cm). Experiment with this range because of the reality you can need a touch more or less. When you discover what works for you, tie off a knot on the factor in which you're conserving the chain, so you don't ought to do this again the following time you operate the pendulum. If it's a string or a cord, you could clearly reduce it off at that factor and then tie a knot.

Yes, No, Maybe

When you've got determined the proper duration, it's time to discern out what your pendulum is making an attempt to inform you. Make positive the pendulum is extraordinary and however first, after which ask it to expose you what a "sure" reaction seems like. It doesn't rely whether or not or no longer or not you ask this query out loud or on your thoughts — both manner, the pendulum will solution you. Keep in mind that it is able to take your pendulum some time before it begins offevolved moving to offer you an answer, but don't worry about that. Just preserve your intention on reading what movement it makes use of to represent "certain," and it is going to begin transferring.

For the maximum detail, humans get outcomes right away, however if it doesn't appear for you on the primary or even 10th try, don't permit that be a reason an excellent manner to stop. You're going to acquire solutions, and once they start coming, they'll get in loads faster and grow to be greater accurate over the years. You need to preserve at this for now not than 5 to 10 minutes every time until it does respond. If the pendulum fails to answer right away, depart it for some moments, re-energize your spirits, and hook up with it again later. After all, you're not a strict lessen-off date!

The pendulum sways back and forth in a clockwise or counterclockwise motion or backward and forward. So, this kind of movements will signal a yes, a no, a in all likelihood, and a fourth alternative, that is "no answer." Chances are this can usually be the way your pendulum answers you, but it doesn't hurt to test earlier than each session to ensure now not something has changed. If checking every consultation feels immoderate, you could do the check sometimes.

Testing Your Pendulum

After you've decided what each motion way, it's time to test the pendulum the usage of actual questions. The high-quality questions to start off with are the ones you recognize the answers to. For instance, you may ask the pendulum:

• Is my call Uncle Sam?

- Did I sincerely have pancakes for breakfast?

- Am I five years antique?

- Do I actually have youngsters?

- Are my eyes on pinnacle of my head?

The idea is surely to ask questions you recognize the answers to so you can be fantastic the entirety works the way it need to. You'll moreover get used to the way your pendulum works within the way. Once you enjoy the pendulum has replied the ones test questions successfully, you can pass right now to asking property you'd like the solution to.

Working with Your Pendulum

Commonly used in divination, pendulums symbolize the cycle of life. They are also a exceptional way of having access to information from your unconscious and the divine nation-states. All you want to do is create a sacred place, floor your self, and follow those steps:

Chapter 23: What Is Lost May Yet Be Found

People lose matters all the time. Sometimes, those subjects are small sufficient that we sincerely shrug and allow them to flow into. Other times, the ones losses can prove very problematic, specifically when the gadgets in query are valuable or high priced to us. It additionally may be quite annoying to recognise you had your glasses excellent a second inside the past, and now for the existence of you, you could't determine out wherein you located them, irrespective of turning your entire residence the other way up. Thankfully, with a pendulum, you don't must

hotel to ransack your property on every occasion you lose some thing.

I've had many opinions in which I'd lose some factor and discover it in a rely of mins in truth running with the pendulum. I'm extremely good you could discover the outcomes you get collectively together with your pendulum as outstanding as many others do. It's a brilliant device for pulling out relevant statistics out of your subconscious mind, this is the a part of you that's aware of in which you dropped your keys or glasses (it is aware of they've been on pinnacle of your head the entire time). The subconscious is privy to all, on the aspect of some of the maximum brilliant assets you had no idea you knew. So, with the pendulum, you may tap into your subconscious mind and retrieve the facts you need. This practical financial ruin is devoted

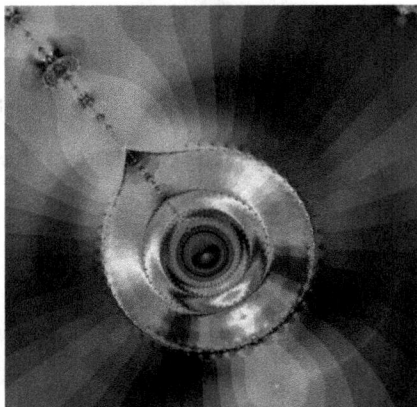

to the use of the power of your pendulum to retrieve lost gadgets.

Relaxation Is Key

When you're searching out some trouble, it's natural which you would probable feel flustered and frustrated. However, it's vital which you make an effort to loosen up in advance than you start asking your pendulum questions, especially in case you need accurate answers. So, for starters, you need to calm your nerves. You can do that by way of the use of using taking a few deep breaths in thru your nostrils, exhaling via slightly parted lips each time. If the exhale is longer than the inhale, that's quality. Don't beat your self up about how deeply or properly you're breathing or how well you time the manner. The purpose is to lighten up. Let circulate of the entirety else and awareness your attention to your respiratory. When you revel in cushty, it's time to ask your pendulum questions about wherein the ones keys are hiding.

Finding What's Lost

The first component is to installation the general region of the thing you're searching out. It in no manner enables to spend your whole time combing thru each room even as it's truely outdoor your property or in a completely unique vicinity absolutely. So, first, you need to reflect onconsideration on wherein you have got been the very last time you saw the item or who handled it remaining and use that to decide out a list of likely regions or places it may be hiding.

• Method 1

Start by way of the use of asking your pendulum a query you recognize the solution to. For example, if you out of place the item inner your home, you could ask whether or now not the object remains in your property, with the expectancy of having a YES. Remember, it's critical which you already be advantageous of the overall place of the object. Despite this, hold your thoughts open for surprises. You might be truly certain it's however in your property, simplest for it to expose out you left it at a chum's or at paintings. In that case, the pendulum ought to obviously solution NO, and it's up to you to artwork your way decrease again to the very last time you found the object, so that you can ask your pendulum if it is probably in a unique region. For the purpose cf this approach, we'll anticipate the item you out of region remains in your own home.

Next, you could ask your pendulum if the object is positioned in a wonderful room. Work your way from one room to the subsequent. While it could not be extraordinary powerful to duplicate the manner with every room, experience unfastened to gather this in case you enjoy the want to. It need to certainly be enough to ask your pendulum, "Is it in the kitchen?" or, "Is it inside the bedroom?" and art work your way through each room in your private home till you get an affirmative solution.

Say the item happens to be within the kitchen, and also you find out there are way too many possible spots in this room wherein you may have lost them. You want to truely ask the pendulum, "Is it inside the left a part of the room?" or "Is it in a cabinet?" If you get a NO, ask if it's within the center component, then the proper element.

Now, it's time to hone in on wherein that object is. You can look at each portion of the distance and ask the pendulum if it is probably there, whether or not or now not that's the desk, drawers, closet, in a laundry pile, underneath your shoes, or anyplace else. Keep going till you discover what you're seeking out – it's certain to expose up somewhere, and your pendulum may be there that will help you all alongside.

- Method 2

Anchor your self in any room of your private home and sit in a snug characteristic. Mentally undergo each room on your thoughts as you watch the manner the pendulum swings. When the pendulum in the end swings YES, as a positive room is in your thoughts, visit that room and continue to be in a single spot. Mentally run via each viable spot within the room as you watch the pendulum swing and wait until you subsequently get a YES. This way, you don't want to invite any questions aloud, and you may artwork for your capability to speak thoughts and transmit energy in your pendulum non-verbally.

- Method 3

Go into the correct room whilst you've narrowed it down, and permit the pendulum to swing to expose you the region of what you've lost. You may also have a study that the nearer you get to the item, the quicker or the slower it's going to drift, counting on how your pendulum is careworn. It's a superb concept to exercise this with an item you may surely see, so that you apprehend how your pendulum responds when you have that object in mind.

Before you search for what's out of location, you can pick out out any random object you notice within the room, repair it for your mind, and notice how your pendulum reacts whilst you get closer to the item (as opposed to even as you skip similarly faraway from it). Then, use this to determine out what the pendulum is attempting to inform you as you get nearer or similarly from the missing item. Another manner the pendulum helps you to recognize in which the misplaced item is by using manner of imparting you with a moderate tug or a jerk. You can also phrase increased anxiety because the pendulum swings.

Connecting with Infinite Intelligence

When seeking out some thing that has been out of place for a long term, chances are you do not have the statistics on in which it could be to your subconscious thoughts. For this cause, it makes revel in to connect with infinite intelligence, that is the intelligence of the universe. This is the intelligence everybody have a connection to – it's the stuff that evokes us all to have first rate thoughts, flashes of concept, bursts of creativity, and more.

So, in case you need to discover some factor you've pretty plenty given up need on finding, you can notwithstanding the truth that do this because of the reality the pendulum will function a connection among you and limitless intelligence, which is aware of in which what you're searching out for can be observed. By asking questions and first rate-tuning them, you'll eventually be capable of locate what you need.

Tips for Looking for Lost Items with Your Pendulum

Let's expect which you've out of place a belt of yours and also you would love to find out it. It may be very useful to have a clean photo of what that belt seems like in your mind. If you aren't the high-quality at visualizing pics for your mind, consider what it appears like on your hands. Everyone has a certain bodily revel in (sight, odor, hearing, flavor, contact) they are capable of replicate of their imagination without problems. So, if sight doesn't be without a doubt proper for you, try any of the opportunity 4. In our example, it wouldn't make experience to need to taste, be aware of, or scent your belt. So, we'll need to art work with each sight or contact, or each if you make a decision upon.

Once you have the picture or sensation of your belt firmly planted to your mind, brazenly ask your pendulum if it is privy to in which to find it. It's additionally an brilliant concept to ask your pendulum whether or not or no longer it's a splendid time to begin seeking out your belt. This is a good query to invite because of the reality you will probable research that it isn't an fantastic time and that your priorities lie some different vicinity.

Perhaps there is probably a few distraction inside the method of your seek which you haven't foreseen.

Another aspect to go through in mind at the same time as performing pendulum searches is that there can be this form of detail as active obstructions. In unique phrases, there might be a few barrier the various object you're searching out and your pendulum that makes it hard for it to spot. Whenever that is the case, you'll have a examine that your pendulum moves in circles instead of presenting you with easy "sure" or "no" solutions. In that situation, all you want to do is modify your position and try asking again. If your pendulum keeps to confuse you, chances are you are not looking within the right area to start with, and you've to test a few region else.

There's not some thing pretty like combining the electricity of a pendulum with a map whilst you're looking for some issue or someone. Maps are focused outlines of geographical places, so it makes it masses much less complicated in your pendulum to pinpoint anything you need. This is to be had in specially useful whilst you are not able to recreate a superb place for your thoughts. If you may get a map this is to scale, even higher. If you can't, you could although paintings with a map app in your cellular telephone or tablet, however possibilities are you will ought to zoom in. When your map is prepared, draw near your pendulum over it and permit it to artwork its magic. If you're searching in a selected building, you may draw the format of that building in vicinity of an real map, so that you can draw close the pendulum over every vicinity and decide out if you have the right room to your missing object or person.

Understanding Why Dowsing May Not Work

As we've described inside the starting monetary disaster, dowsing is a divination technique used to discover radiations emitted from all topics spherical us. At instances, no matter our maximum valiant efforts to discover an object the use of the dowsing approach, it seems to maintain no tangible outcomes. . There are several opportunities as to why you're no longer having any fulfillment with the technique. For one, you could have a completely sturdy attachment to the results. If this is the case, you need to find out a way to detach your self out of your expectancies to permit the dowsing to take location because it need to. Remember, this is not about controlling what the pendulum does, however alternatively, permitting it to show you what your unconscious and endless intelligence are telling you.

Chapter 24: Better Health with the Pendulum

"Health is wealth," goes the popular announcing. Before I move any similar y into this financial disaster, I need to make some thing in truth easy. You need to make sure which you reap out to the proper experts to get looked at if you are experiencing any issues together with your fitness, whether or not bodily or highbrow. Do no longer leap to conclusions or make crucial assumptions based totally totally on what your pendulum tells. While it could serve to guide your non secular recognition and increase, the pendulum should in no way be taken into consideration a opportunity for proper medical recommendation and diagnosis from a certified fitness professional. With that being said, permit's discover how you can achieve higher health way to the power of the pendulum.

History of Pendulum Magic in Medicine and Health

The use of pendulums in treatment may be traced back as a ways as 500 B.C in Ancient Greece, when Hippocrates, a famend medical physician, and philosopher, wrote approximately the usage of pendulums in remedy. Traditionally taken into consideration the "father of cutting-edge remedy," he moreover actual one-of-a-type strategies which includes draining blood with leeches, cupping (the use of cups on sufferers' pores and pores and pores and skin), and administering ointments.

Hippocrates himself wrote about pendulums with the first-rate regard. In his writings, he mentioned the manner it modified into vital to hold one's thoughts targeted on the venture at hand, in any other case divine solutions or recovery may also now not come for a affected character. He additionally said the importance of preserving both fingers consistent and no longer touching the pendulum in any manner, as "that is a factor which has been left out via the use of many; most people contact their pendulum and consequently make themselves worried." Hippocrates' hobby at the purity of a affected man or woman's u.S. Of the usa of mind and body endorsed later uses of pendulums for recuperation functions.

During the Middle Ages, numerous physicians went on to perpetuate Hipprocrates' legacy approximately pendulums and used them for their private features. Galen, a clinical physician, and fact seeker in Ancient Rome, wrote a treatise on the use of pendulums. His writings verify using pendulums in remedy and art work at some point of the Roman technology. He states that the most crucial of these practices problem the remedy of illnesses and preventing bleeding by way of a small spherical board hung earlier than the affected individual's bed. Galen moreover confirms that sufferers used pendulums for clinical functions all through his time.

Pliny mentions its use a number of the Romans as well. They would take a small spherical or oval piece of timber, place the photograph of an animal on it, and song every direction of the pendulum's swing – if those guides coincided with the herbal symptoms, you can have a successful therapy.

Dioscorides, a Greek doctor, and creator who lived within the 1st century A.D., moreover wrote about the pendulum as a tool for treating contamination. He described how pendulums may be used to diagnose ailments, characterize the time of day, and useful useful useful resource within the remedy of illnesses with the resource of "looking the upward push and fall with attention."

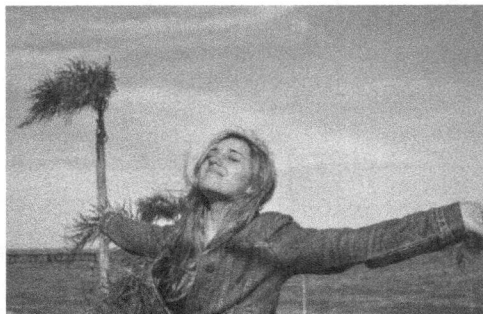

Claudius Galenus' writings additionally illustrate using pendulums to diagnose numerous sicknesses. He wrote about how the Ancient Greeks can also want to use a small live with a carved image on it to symbolize part of the frame, then keep the stick from a string and take a look at the way it moved. If the stick moved in an normal manner, it meant there has been a few factor incorrect with the a part of the body represented on the wooden carving.

Pendulums continued to be used medically afterward, as evidenced in spiritual books from the tenth to the 16th century. For instance, John of Mirfield, a 13th-century English monk, wrote at length about the medicinal programs of the pendulum. The affected character might probable have a string tied to their left hand with the pendulum on it and can swing it up and down over a basin of water until they have been healed.

Numerous paintings have been discovered that display how humans used pendulums as equipment for healing. Notably, a portray decided inside the Vatican inside the 1500s depicts a nun (Maria de Azevedo) using two small wooden bowls that resemble pendulums to diploma the blood strain of a affected individual.

The use of pendulums survived well into the twentieth century as well, with many clinical doctors and researchers locating strategies to decorate their accuracy. The most commonplace method changed into to hang them on strings that would spin in 3 exceptional strategies: clockwise, counter-clockwise, or at unique speeds. In 1867, an English health practitioner named Stephen O'Connor used a pendulum to determine the right treatment time body for sufferers who suffered complications throughout surgical treatment.

In the nineteenth century, French Surgeon General Hocquard used a pendulum in a way known as "location treatment" to diagnose illnesses. This became a famous technique in a few unspecified time within the destiny of the 1920s and Thirties. In 1964, Charles de Lacey, a French ear fitness care expert, determined that if one ought to change the pitch of the string, they might alternate the fee at which it would swing. By changing the rate at which he swung his pendulum, he changed into able to write down what prompted a selected pitch with tremendous swings of his pendulum. For instance, he determined that tone A produced a to-and-fro of over 6 inches, at the same time as tone E produced a to-and-fro of inches. He used this discovery to discover what ailments have been associated with wonderful tones.

Another character who researched this modified into Dr. Nilsson, a well-known Swedish ethnologist who used pendulums for research purposes in recuperation. In 1945, he wrote about how superb tones may be obtained from the pendulum the use of vocal cords and vowel sounds. Through using his pendulum on human beings or businesses, he additionally found that some human beings replied in any other case to certain tones acquired from the pendulum than others did. He believed his pendulum become a way of finding out facts about beyond lives as properly. Dr. Nilsson stated, "It is consequently possible for someone to 'undergo in thoughts' certain statistics belonging to a former life on this planet or activities belonging to a miles off destiny." While this ought to be interested in a grain of salt, his discoveries aspect to the awesome scientific ability of pendulums.

In 1975, William Nelson cautioned the pendulum may be used as a diagnostic device because it detected disturbances within the frame's electromagnetic area. According to him, the electromagnetic area modified right into a "herbal strain that continues the entirety in stability." He based totally his concept on the art work of Dr. Wilhelm Reich, who felt that, all through orgasm, humans's electric powered fee may be disrupted and that this disturbance may want to result in ailments. Nelson additionally asserted that the use of a pendulum may want to assist come across sick factors of the human frame.
A Quick Test

If you need to discover firsthand whether or no longer a pendulum may be useful as a diagnostic device, there's a easy test you can do proper now. First, take a seat in a snug function, and permit the pendulum to hold over your thigh. Let it swing as you area the cause to discover whether or not or not the pores and pores and skin of your thigh is terrific. (This check presupposes there's not something incorrect in conjunction with your pores and pores and skin right here, however if there can be, you could virtually artwork with any other wholesome a part of your body permit your pendulum to hold over it.) Your pendulum want to swing YES, telling you that it's in reality exceptional.

Next, pinch your thigh brilliant and difficult so that it stings you substantially, but not so difficult which you damage your pores and skin. Now, allow the pendulum to swing over this pinched pores and skin, and be conscious the pendulum as it begins to swing proper away within the NO direction. Allow the pendulum to understand over this patch of pores and pores and skin as you continue to maintain the cause of locating out in case you're terrific – you'll be conscious that because the ache is going away, your pendulum will slowly shift from swinging NO to YES, telling you that your pores and pores and skin has recovered.

Similarly, you could carry out this diagnostic test each time you feel there's a few component off along with your body and you need to pinpoint the precise problem place to allow your medical physician recognize about it.

Pendulum Magic for Energetic Health

Chakras are an historic concept determined in lots of religions and religious beliefs. Essentially, chakras are electricity centers that govern numerous factors of your body's organic abilities, together with health and homeostasis (in one of a kind terms, the body's capability to self-regulate). This concept is most often associated with Eastern cultures and non secular structures, however Western spiritualists have used the pendulum for hundreds of years.

By using their pendulum to art work thru their non-public chakra tool, spiritualists can stability out the energies internal themselves. You can gather the equal with the aid of following the ones steps:

1.   Decide on a body detail in that you want to begin operating collectively along with your

pendulum. This may be your sun plexus, coronary coronary heart, or 0.33 eye area – everywhere to your body in which you experience an strength imbalance. The seven fundamental chakras you may artwork on are: the premise, sacral, solar plexus, coronary coronary heart, throat, 0.33 eye, and crown chakras. More statistics can be provided on what the ones chakras have an effect on, so you apprehend the varieties of questions you need to invite yourself to analyze the manner you may carry them again into balance.

2.   Formulate a clean query for your self based mostly on what chakra you're running with. This may be some detail as simple as "Does my coronary coronary heart chakra need balancing?" or "Is my solar plexus chakra in stability?" Keep the ones questions easy and intuitive to keep a slim, well-described interest.

3.   Hold your pendulum over the region of your deciding on. Make first rate the chain is stretched sufficient to wherein it could start shifting. You will understand at the same time as it is stretched sufficient whilst all of the

energy starts flowing freely through it, and you feel a subtle energy shift internal your body.

4.   Ask yourself more questions depending on what you get as an answer. For example, you will be extra unique in case you find out your coronary heart chakra is out of stability via manner of asking, "Is it due to the fact there's a few element or someone I can't forgive?" or "Is this block because of fear?" If the solution is YES, you could get even extra particular. You by myself recognize precisely what you need to ask.

five.   Now, permit pass of the pendulum. When you have got were given were given your solutions, start activating your chakra's energies and notice the way you revel in. You can try this mentally through envisioning that chakra being charged with radiant white slight or a light that suits its color. Alternatively, sense the chakras themselves simply via sitting along with your eyes near as you breathe. Envision your breath moving into through the chakra that needs balancing, and that as you exhale, it feels higher and clearer.

Get a feel of the strength your chakras are generating, in which they may be positioned for your frame, and the manner they are responding to being activated. Repeat this each time you experience drawn to start going for walks collectively along with your chakras – try this as quickly as, instances, or 3 instances a day. At the identical time, make sure to preserve your pendulum near you always. This lets in you to apply it for other matters in your every day lifestyles as well, which incorporates asking questions about humans and gadgets round you.

After doing this some instances, you can begin to get a better revel in for a manner the ones specific chakras must enjoy for your frame. This makes it a whole lot less hard for you to tell if they're balanced or not, absolutely through asking your self, "How does this feel?" or "How can I make this strength higher?"

What You Need to Know approximately Chakras

In this devoted phase, we're going to take a higher check the seven chakras so that you can decide out the manner to paintings along with your pendulum to hold balance to all elements of your electricity body. As you find out the tendencies of every fundamental chakra, you'll bring yourself one step in the direction of the non secular success you're trying to find in enhancing your existence.

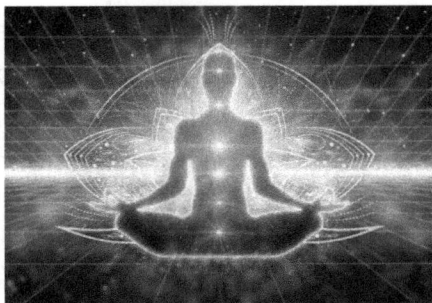

First of all, the foundation chakra, referred to as the muladhara, sits at the bottom of your backbone. It's the basis of life that brings stability and balance within the complete problem, even at the same time as you're faced with difficult demanding situations. When it's balanced, you experience solid in yourself. Blockages in this chakra take region for your bodily lifestyles as foot and leg ache, disturbance at home, feeling insecure and inadequate, excessive strain, sluggishness, and regression. Stones you could use to rebalance this chakra are pink jasper, hematite, and garnet.

The sacral chakra is called the svadhisthana. It's located proper above the inspiration chakra, slightly under your stomach button. It's all about your sexual and cutting-edge lifestyles, and it's the purpose you can hook up with your emotional self and have interaction with others on an emotional level. Whenever you look at you're not allowing yourself to revel in, that you could't bear in thoughts or create effectively, otherwise you enjoy you're overwhelmed with too many feelings or don't just like the manner you appearance, that may be a signal that this chakra have to use some balancing. Physical imbalance signs and symptoms and symptoms on this chakra embody pain on your lower returned and hips. Use amber and carnelian to balance this one.

The solar plexus chakra is the manipura. It's located to your stomach, and it's the motive you revel in self perception and vanity. When there's a balance right here, you experience together with you're on top of factors. By comparison, while it's out of stability, you may enjoy issues with digestion and stomach ache, you overvalue your ego, and might't take rate on your relationships. You may additionally moreover enjoy like you have not any electricity, which you have commitment troubles and feature trouble seeing your plans thru. Tiger's eye, agate, yellow jade, and citrine are the notable stones to heal this chakra.

Chapter 25: Pendulum Protection

The root of the whole thing in life is religious. With the pendulum, you can expect to analyze plenty more about the world of spirit as you hook up with your subconscious and countless intelligence. Thanks to the pendulum, you'll be able to art work with energies other humans do now not be privy to or barely choose out out up on, the subtle energies we use in manifestation, safety, restoration, and similarly. Let's find out how you can use the pendulum to artwork with the spirit for one of a kind dreams.

Unintentional Evil

The factor approximately magic is it may be used for wonderful or evil. There are those who are looking for for to harm others via running dark magic, and for this reason, it's clever to comprehend a way to shield your self from those non secular and psychic attacks. Just as it's far viable to exercise recuperation humans at a distance, it's miles feasible to influence people negatively from afar. Generally speaking, in case you don't intend damage to every body and a person tries to curse you, the spell will haven't any choice however to transport back to the sender. For the maximum issue, practitioners of magic recognize it's far unethical to cause others harm. However, that doesn't propose you shouldn't be capable of shield yourself from lousy juju.

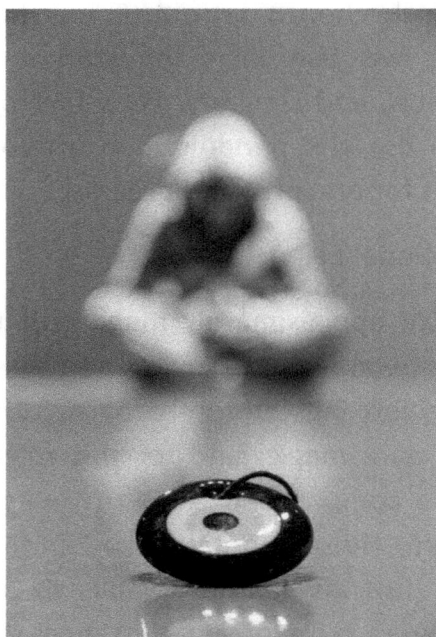

Another problem approximately non secular and psychic attacks is they're not usually deliberate. Remember how I talked about idea bureaucracy? Think approximately others and awful processes, but they don't realize how a whole lot damage they are causing. Then, there are folks which might be power vampires but do not understand it. Energy vampires find out they'll restore their strength stages through leaching distinct humans's. The presence of an energy vampire appears like you're inexplicably tired, not truly physical however mentally and spiritually as properly. It's typically a comfort to stroll a long way from their employer. They understand if you have honestly nicely power and also you're feeling your brilliant — because of the reality that's after they want to come back round you and drain you.

You need to understand which you do not owe all of us electricity. You don't have to remain of their presence for longer than important. At any time, you have were given the proper to stroll away from situations and people that do not go away you feeling proper or assist you recharge yourself. Again, hold in mind that a number of the ones human beings aren't even consciously aware of what they're doing, so don't skip spherical wondering the worst of them due to the truth that would most effective motive more damage. Always stay proper to yourself, pontificate amazing feature, and desire others well.

Checking In with Your Pendulum

Make it a detail to check in together with your pendulum each every so often to find out if an strength vampire became draining you. If you're having a conversation with a person, you can step away momentarily to can use your pendulum and check on the electricity of the person you're talking with. Of route, you don't need to do that with simply all of us because that might genuinely make subjects weird. Some of the signs you will probably phrase on the identical time as you're being worn-out or harmed by using way of manner of a person includes experiencing a stunning drop in power and feeling inexplicably fatigued, even in case you've had a few fantastic sleep and generally cope with your self. Another manner to inform you're underneath psychic and spiritual attack is which you'll be predisposed to have brilliant nightmares. You might also have habitual desires, irrespective of what you do. It appears as even though your mind is decided to playback those equal scenes over and over every night time time.

Other symptoms embody experiencing all styles of bodily hassle together along with your body while you know you're usually healthful and in form. Likewise, if you note topics spherical you begin breaking down, that you constantly find out your self in accidents, or that horrific data begin to flow to you quicker than regular, those may be symptoms which you are being spiritually or psychically attacked, intentionally or no longer. You may additionally additionally moreover phrase that you no longer care approximately existence collectively with you used to and may also be teetering on the brink of depression.

Now, this is not to insinuate that each time you experience depressed, it is due to the truth you are psychically and spiritually attacked. Check in with a expert therapist that will help you parent out whether or not or now not the problem can be bodily. That stated, when you have no records of persistent despair or unique highbrow health conditions, it is able to be a inform-story signal which you're under assault.

Keeping music of your self spiritually, mentally, and bodily is essential. So, every time some problem appears off, you may check alongside facet your pendulum and find out if that's simply the case. You also can use your pendulum to ask exactly what's causing it and the way you can recuperation it. For example, if you're a workaholic constantly immersed in paintings, in no manner permitting your self to relaxation among tasks, it's splendid natural that you start to experience overwhelming pressure. The extra stressed you're, the more your physical fitness might be affected in one-of-a-type tactics. When this is the case, you have to determine out what to do to heal your self. However, if you understand which you are able to dealing with the quantity of exertions you typically do, then you definitely definately definately may probable need to check in collectively along with your pendulum. It can let you recognise that you are absolutely being attacked energetically.

Unmasking Your Enemies

The pendulum can do hundreds greater than actually telling you what the hassle is. If it seems you are in fact, being attacked, your pendulum can allow you to realize who is responsible. The humorous thing approximately existence is that you're busy going approximately your company, and a person else has lots of hate or jealousy for you of their coronary heart. Also, it's possible that you could have angry a person without even understanding it. You also can be attacked through a being that doesn't exist on the bodily plane. With these type of alternatives in thoughts, you should ask your pendulum the right questions to determine out the premise deliver and examine who is inflicting you such harm.

Bespoke Protection

It's no longer sufficient to apprehend who's answerable for your dilemmas in existence.

The greater crucial question is, how do you shield your self from those poor energies? There's no better manner than to test in with your pendulum. Generally talking, as long as you keep a incredible thoughts-set and a coronary heart full of love, there may be no manner the ones assaults can be sustained. More often than not, what keeps the ones attacks going is your thoughts-set and mind-set towards them. If you're constantly mired in worry and sadness, it actually feeds that strength even more and makes you continue to experience worse and worse sports. You have to generally preserve in mind that the pleasant way you can ever be harmed is if you do not forget you could be harmed, and if you trust which you do want to be heard. Optimism and self-self perception are the first rate defenses in opposition to unfriendly, negative magic.

Fortunately, tremendous practices can help boom your non secular power, despite the fact that you have to not interact in them until you accept as true with in them wholeheartedly. So, as continuously, keep an open thoughts. You should ask your pendulum if this is a matter you want to wish approximately if you receive as actual with within the strength of prayer. If you are a religious man or woman who believes within the power of fasting, you may test in along with your pendulum to appearance if that's the extraordinary direction of motion for this problem. Regardless of the scenario, always take a look at in with a systematic expert earlier than you embark on such non secular practices as fasting, to ensure you're not harming your health in the approach Here are some questions you can need to invite your pendulum:

•	Do I want to do something to make this save you?

•	Should I pray approximately this situation?

•	Will fasting kind the whole lot out?

•	Do I need to soak up a few distinctive shape of meditation?

•	If I acquire out to this character to express regret, will the assaults prevent?

- Do I need to enhance my air of mystery? Will that be enough?

We all have natural safety in opposition to awful electricity. This safety is referred to as your air of mystery. It is the number one barrier that everybody who wants to motive you to damage will want to penetrate. Just like any other shape of safety, you may make more potent it. Here are some smooth practices you may carry out to expand a more potent air of thriller this is proof in opposition to all sorts of attacks:

1. Meditation: Find a pleasing and quiet place wherein you may not be disturbed for at least 10 to 15 mins. Make superb you're sporting cushty apparel. It needs to be free, so you don't feel like every part of it is defensive without delay to you uncomfortably. You can sit down down on a chair, or on the floor in the Lotus function if you select out. If it helps, use a yoga mat. You want to discover a chair or table wherein you can set your forearm down and permit your pendulum to recognise within the direction of the ground as you carry out this workout.

Shut your eyes and take a deep breath n thru your nostril. Hold that breath for a few moments, experience it sit down down inside you, and lightly breathe it via your barely parted lips. Now you're going to breathe in all over again, and as you do, bear in mird that your air of thriller is a strong white slight that emanates from the middle of your being and truely surrounds your complete body. Feel the overall of lifestyles warmth and energy of the charisma as it glows all round you. As you exhale yet again, photograph your air of mystery developing stronger and large. You have your pendulum for your hand tc assist you to understand how strong your air of mystery is. Depending on how your perdulum is programmed, your air of thriller strength will be proven as both dramatic motion or a whole and utter stillness of the pendulum. This will will let you recognize which you have reinforced your air of thriller sufficiently.

2.   Get Some Air and Light: Have ycu ever walked right into a room that didn't gather any glowing air or received any mild in a long time? Apart from the musty scent and the damp   feeling,   you   may   moreover   be

conscious the room feels oppressive and is complete of dark, horrible strength. You're no longer imagining this. The equal trouble can show up to you whilst you're continuously cooped up indoors, and also you don't permit your self to get any solar or easy air. Make it a addiction of going out ordinary, even for a couple of minutes, so you can recharge your body and rid yourself of horrible energies which have accrued over the years.

The solar is splendid as it will feed every chakra for your frame, each main and minor, strengthening your air of mystery and making it really impermeable to the forces of evil. Take a conscious 2d to respire deeply and permit the air rejuvenate your spirits from internal on every occasion you're outside. Disconnect for a right away. Appreciate those moments of reference to yourself and nature. Let them encourage you to spend greater time out of doors, under the solar's recovery powers. Now that you've spent some time taking in that adorable air and light, you solicit your pendulum to discover whether or not or now not or now not your air of thriller is adequately sturdy. Ask if spending time out of doors is enough to cleanse you of all the horrific energy you've been wearing.

three.   Move Your Body: You need to each take a stroll, exercising, or have someone provide you with a rub down. Staying physical lively will help split any bad air of thriller and allow your energies to drift another time. Before deciding on the way you need to glide your body, check in with the pendulum to look what have to serve you the tremendous. Sure, you're going to get results from some element you decide, but it's great to go along with what you need at that unique point in time.

4.   Laugh Deliberately: Laughter is one of the maximum super treatments, and what human beings don't recognize is laughter can be a exceptional way to take area your desires. The vibration of laughter is so immoderate and herbal that it cannot be brought down with the useful resource of way of some thing under it. Here's a fascinating issue you may no longer be aware about: You do not need a purpose to chortle.

You can simply pick out to chortle your head off for a minute or two after which take note of the shift in energies from in advance than you commenced out and once you're finished guffawing. Make it a point to look at comedies, check humorous subjects, and usually search for the hilarious perspective to every experience in lifestyles.

Some people are inherently capable of laughing no matter how horrible a state of affairs they're going thru, and that's due to the truth they've selected to stay excellent in the face of adversity. Not all of them are psychopaths, despite the fact that. Laughter works for putting off all topics negative. So, the following time you feel unhappy or down, otherwise you're experiencing what you located might be a highbrow or non secular attack toward you, you need to don't forget giggling it out. It may also moreover moreover simply deliver the comfort you're searching for in the ones tough times.